Underneath the SCARS

CANDIDA SULLIVAN

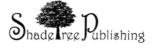

Underneath the Scars

By Candida Sullivan
Copyright @ 2011 ShadeTree Publishing, LLC
1038 N. Eisenhower Dr. #274
Beckley, West Virginia 25801
ISBN: 978-1-937331-04-7
Printed in the United States of America

Scripture quotations are taken from the King James Version, which is public domain in the United States.

All rights reserved. This book is protected by copyright. No part of this book may be reproduced or transmitted in any form or by any means, electronic or mechanical, including photocopying, recording, or by any information storage and retrieval system, without permission in writing from the publisher.

The purpose of this book is to educate and enlighten. This book is sold with the understanding that the publisher and author are not engaged in rendering counseling, albeit it professional or lay, to the reader or anyone else. The author shall have neither liability nor responsibility to any person or entity with respect to any loss or damage caused, or alleged to have been caused, directly or indirectly, by the information contain in this book.

Visit our Web site at www.ShadeTreePublishing.com

Thank you God for giving me life and showing me I did have a beautiful story to tell!

To my Mom and Dad. Thank you for loving me just as I am and for never trying to change me. Thank you for always encouraging me and for teaching me that with God anything is possible.

To my family and friends, thank you for NEVER giving up on me!

CONTENTS

INTRODUCTION 1
A Prayer and a Dream 5
As One Door Closes, Another One Opens........................11
The Diagnosis 19
Answers to the Future Often Lie in the Past....................25
Learning to Overcome Obstacles 33
Heartaches and Fears..41
Blinded by Scars..47
Confidence is Earned..57
The Fairy Tale 61
Tolerance is not Acceptance 69
Stares and Smiles 75
Out of the Mouths of Kids 81
Ability in Disability..87
The Choice to be Happy 91
Mold Me Lord 95
Trusting the Lord...99
FOR KIDS..103
ABOUT AMNIOTIC BAND SYNDROME........107
ACKNOWLEDGEMENTS 109
ABOUT THE AUTHOR...111

INTRODUCTION

When I was a little girl, I prayed the same prayer every night. I kneeled down, clasped my scarred hands, and begged God to heal them. I wanted him to take away my scars, and I believed in my heart He could heal me, just as He had healed the people in the Bible. Then I could proclaim His healing power, just as they had.

Every morning, I would open my eyes with hope dancing in my heart. I would inhale deeply and jerk my hands out from underneath the covers, expecting the big voilà, but it never happened. Thoroughly disappointed, every day, I would wonder what I had done wrong. Why wouldn't God answer my prayer?

I hated being different. People frequently laughed, starred, and teased me, if not verbally then with their expressions. Then the big question was always asked, "What happened to your hands?" The questioned bothered me almost as much as the scars themselves because I didn't have an explanation to satisfy their interest. Saying, "I was born this way" didn't appease their curiosity any more than it did my own. Every time I delivered my inadequate explanation I received the standard, "Oh you poor thing, bless your little heart." And that made me feel worse. It was as if I was cursed – forced to bear the scars of disgrace.

I often wished for some elaborate story that would turn my ugly scars into something beautiful. I wanted a story filled with inspiration that would turn the pity in their eyes to awe. Somehow, I thought the story behind the scars would change the way others looked at me.

Underneath the Scars

Some called it a fluke of nature, while others wondered how God could to do that to a child. I, however, thought it was unfair. We only get one life to live and I am forced to live my life burdened with scars as ugly as the way others treated me.

Growing up, I wasn't a normal child. I didn't think the way other children typically think. I always wanted to be older; somehow I thought when I grew up that people would stop being cruel. Instead of dreaming about childish things (like toys, playing, etc.); I dreamed of Heaven. I knew that when I went to Heaven I wouldn't be scarred anymore. I would look like the angels and I was absolutely positive they were perfect. Sometimes I would imagine what my hands would look like if they were perfect. How would they feel? How great would it be to actually be able to do whatever I wanted without limitations?

I wanted someone to look at me and, for once, think I was beautiful. I wanted to be normal and I tried so hard to prove that I could do anything that everyone else could do. I quickly learned that regardless of my accomplishments and strength, no one would ever look at me as just an ordinary person.

To some I was disabled, to others I was handicapped. Some thought I was special, while others shared my assumption that I was indeed cursed. Even when some people praised me for my accomplishments, it would be like - that's great you were able to do that with your handicap.

But there comes a point in everyone's life where a decision must be made - live or merely exist. It was apparent that God was not going to heal my hands. I could A) wallow in self-pity for the rest of my life, B) live in the shadows of life, or C) while I would never be ordinary, I could strive to be extraordinary.

In my mind, I never believed I would ever become an extraordinary person, but it felt amazing to allow myself to dream. I think dreams have a lyrical charm that are both comforting and inspiring. They challenge us all to rise above the rumble and proclaim we are alive. They force us to look by faith, past the tangible things we can hold and see, and hope for the desires of our hearts. The real dreams are the ones that seem so impossible, but through faith, courage, and determination become possible.

My life really started with a prayer and a dream. And God did answer my prayer – He healed my scars through my dreams. Only it wasn't exactly the way I had intended. My journey to acceptance wasn't easy. It was a battle every step of the way; but oh, what a journey it has been.

My life is neither heroic nor exciting; I'm neither wealthy nor famous. Nevertheless, God has blessed me with a beautiful story. If you skimmed the surface of my life, it would probably appear dull, but I don't think anyone would call it normal. I can't say that I've suffered. I have had trials and tribulations as well as numerous obstacles to overcome.

I eventually discovered the cause of my scars. Amniotic Band Syndrome (ABS) is a rare condition caused by string-like bands in the amniotic sac. These bands can entangle the umbilical cord or other parts of the baby's body. The constriction can cause a variety of problems depending on where they are located and how tightly they are wrapped. The complications from ABS vary. In my case, the banding had resulted in amputation and scarring on several places of my body.

ABS not only affects my hands, foot, and arm, but also it affects every aspect of my life. And that is what I want to share with you: my feelings, trials and tribulations, accomplishments and failures, fears and courage, disappointments and hope. I want to show you how a different perspective on life can, in all reality, change your life too. Through it all, I have learned that I am not a victim, but a survivor!

Some of the words will be hard for you to read - they were hard for me to write. There's a little voice inside my head that continues to tell me that if I write about God and mention Him too often, no one will want to read my story, but if I remove God, then I have nothing

I've tried to write this story as honestly as possible from my heart without exaggerating or making something seem beautiful that was really ugly. I've tried to take myself back to those moments of my life when the events happened, and tried to write from the heart of the person who experienced them, not the person I am today. I hope this book helps you in some small way, just as it has helped me.

—Candida Sullivan

Chapter One

A Prayer and a Dream

There are many devices in a man's heart; nevertheless the counsel of the LORD, that shall stand.
            -Proverbs 19:21

    After watching Dr. Phil for years, I've learned that we have defining moments in our lives that bring forth change. For me, it was when I realized there was something missing from my life. I had a wonderful family, a house love had made a home, and in essence, all of my needs were supplied. Nevertheless, the feelings deep down in my heart, that something was missing, burdened me daily.

    I hated my job. There were no wow moments or feelings of accomplishment. I did the job that I was hired and expected to do, and even if I exceeded their expectations, there were no special rewards. When I clocked out every day, I felt as if I had somehow cheated myself and lost eight hours of my life.

    I began searching my heart for the answers. What in the world did Candida Sullivan want to be when she grew up? I couldn't pinpoint the exact career I wanted, but I knew I wanted to help people. I craved a job that would allow me to touch another life - regardless of how big or small. Even though it appeared I had everything, I still lacked the heart of it all. In truth, I wanted to make a difference.

Underneath the Scars

I wondered how others found their special calling in life. Some people always seem to know what they want to do with their lives. It seems they never struggle and always find the right balance of success. How do they know for sure? How do they know when they enter college that they will love the career they have chosen?

I thought about teaching because I loved kids and challenges. I loved seeing the flicker of understanding and amazement on their faces. Maybe that was my special gift - to love and teach children. It was exciting to contemplate.

The stars quickly fizzled out of my eyes and the reality appeared. In order to be a teacher, I needed a degree, and the only way to achieve a degree was to attend college. Therefore, I would be forced to quit my fulltime job, still pay for daycare for my child, and somehow afford tuition without getting a foreclosure in the mail.

It seemed hopeless until someone mentioned an organization for the handicapped that would help me with college. I debated the issue for a few months. Each time I came up with the same answer, I wasn't handicapped! How would I be able to look anyone in the eye and admit I was handicapped - when I had spent my entire life trying to prove otherwise? Not to mention, I would be forced to look at myself in the mirror daily.

The long list of reasons to reject the idea outweighed the reasons to accept; yet, the one major reason smiled at me daily, my little boy. I wanted him to look at me with adoration in his eyes. I wanted to be a mommy who he could be proud of, with a special job that actually affected other people's lives. I wanted to be invited to career day, but first I needed a career instead of job.

Once my mind was made up, I went forward without looking back. I will never forget how I felt when I sat in the room with the counselor. I felt as if I were doing something wrong, like I was somewhere I shouldn't have been, and any moment someone would walk in and catch me. Every time I thought about how I would answer the questions, I was sure to be asked, my heart ached and I felt defeated. How was I supposed to say those three words? How could I so openly admit to being disabled, when I had tried my whole life to prove I was able? How could I look her in the eye and say, "I am handicapped?"

Every time I opened my mouth the words stuck in my throat, the tears burned my eyes, and the lie forming on my tongue felt as if it would scorch it. Regardless of how I tried, I couldn't bring myself to say it. Instead, I told her of my fears and how I worried that without a college education I couldn't provide for my child, should something happen to my husband.

I was required to take a test to analyze my disabilities. I knew that I held my own future in my hands. I had the ability to flunk the test, but not the heart. That day I was so afraid. What if when they looked at me through a microscope they saw that I was truly disabled? What if they opened my eyes and showed me I had no chance of success?

As I took the test, my fears were all there guiding and pushing me to do my best. Even though my heart ached and I wanted to protest, I complied with every aspect of the test. It was nothing like I expected. I figured I would be asked to write or take a typing test to truly analyze the use of my hands. In my opinion, the test was unfair to me. I was asked to walk, pick up heavy things; overall, my mobility was tested. There was a single test that evaluated coordination with my hands, but that was it. It was nothing like the rigorous test previous employers had given me.

When the test concluded, the doctor was amazed. Even without surgery or therapy I could use my hands, very well. He assured me – in both his professional and personal opinion – I would be a wonderful teacher.

I waited for my official results with mixed feelings. The price for a degree suddenly seemed too high. Would I ever be able to look at myself the same way again? I felt like I had somehow sold myself short. I had tried to justify my reasons, but still there was no justification. Proclaiming one minute I was not handicapped and then, suddenly, changing my mind to suite my own purposes was wrong. I realized I couldn't sit on both sides of the fence. I was trying to take the easy way out.

It was as if I were asking the government to pay me for my scars. Like I thought they owed me something. My hands had never prevented me from working. It wasn't like my scars prevented me from finding a job. Now if I had previously had a job and then had an accident, or my condition worsened, and I needed assistance to find a job I could perform with my new limitations—that would be different. However, that wasn't my case. I wanted an education because I didn't like my job.

To claim that I wanted to have a special career for my child was absurd. Yes, I wanted him to be proud of me one day, but the journey to the career was just as important as the career itself. Would he or anyone else be proud of the fact that I had pretended to be handicapped for the purpose of personal gain? Okay, so I never came right out and said it, but the fact that I was there insinuated I believed I deserved compensation.

By the time my test results arrived, I no longer cared what the State of Tennessee thought. I knew in my heart I wasn't handicapped. Still my hands trembled as I opened the letter.

According to the results, I was **ABOVE** average on most of the test. Because of the appearance of my hands, my name waits on a long list that will never be called. They will never pay for my college education because of my strong work history and the test results. Even though I'm sure I wouldn't have accepted the money, I'm so thankful God removed the temptation.

As I held the results in my hands, the feeling was bitter sweet; bitter because I knew I couldn't afford to go back to college; and thus, I knew that I would never be a teacher. I was right back to square one, still trying to figure out what to do with my life. The sweet part, however, was that all of my hard work, throughout my life, had paid off. Maybe my quest to being extraordinary wasn't so farfetched after all. If nothing else, it helped me to keep going and try different things.

I tried several more possibilities to find a career, but nothing panned out. It seemed every door I tried to open slammed shut in my face. Finally weak, tired, and afraid, I bowed my head and prayed. I asked God to give me something, anything that would be mine and bless me to help others. After I poured my heart out, I got up off my knees and felt it would all work out.

Underneath the Scars

Chapter Two

As One Door Closes, Another One Opens

Behold, I stand at the door, and knock: if any man hear my voice, and open the door, I will come in to him, and will sup with him, and he with me.

-Revelation 3:20

    I continued my quest to find a career. I inquired about help wanted ads, searched the classifieds, and became a frequent visitor of the employment office. Even though the possibility of a college education had passed, for the time being anyway, still I needed a change or new direction. I went to several interviews, yet nothing panned out.

    I shortly discovered that I was expecting our second child. It just made sense for me to stay where I was because I didn't need the added stress of finding a career, while I was nurturing a new life.

    My second pregnancy was nothing like the first one. I was sick from the moment of conception, and my back ached a few months into the second trimester. My little one decided at six months he wanted to be born, and we used therapy to try and convince him to wait a little longer. At the same time, we found out my papaw had cancer. The struggle inside me was anticipating life, and my papaw was struggling against death. Because of my condition, I took an early maternity leave and spent more time in Kentucky with my family.

Underneath the Scars

Three weeks before my due date, my second son came into the world in a hurry. It was as if he had an appointment to keep. Since everyday was precious and numbered, I went to see my papaw the day after I got home from the hospital. He held my baby in his arms and with tears in his eyes told me he was the prettiest baby he had ever seen. Even though he had seven children of his own, and many grandchildren as well as great grandchildren, I understood what he was saying- this would be the last baby he would ever see or hold.

A few days later, my papaw slipped into a coma and I never got to really talk to him again. He died a few weeks later. It made me think about time and that everything happens for a reason. If I had my baby when he was actually due, my papaw would have never seen him. Had I not have had a complicated pregnancy, then I wouldn't have taken an early maternity leave nor got to spend so many wonderful days by his side.

When my papaw passed away, the grief consumed me. I felt so alone. My papaw and I shared a special bond, even though we never spoke about it. His hand was injured in the war. Three of his fingers had been shot off and his hand attached to his belly for a time. His hand held scars similar to my own. But when he died, I felt more different than I had ever felt before.

Standing beside his coffin, I looked down and noticed his hand showing. Although, the funeral home had initially hidden his hand, my family made them change it - they said he had never hidden or been ashamed of his hand before, and they wouldn't allow it to be portrayed at his death either.

A lump eased into my throat. Why hadn't he been ashamed? Why hadn't he ever tried to hide his hand? Didn't anyone ever stare at him? Of course they did. They had to. But, why didn't it bother him? I suddenly wished I had asked him those questions, but the answers were now buried, and I would never know.

It bothered more than ever that I was still so self-conscious. I wished for some elaborate story to tell others. I wished I felt about my scars the way my papaw had felt. His scars had a purpose, and yet, mine were unknown.

I continued to grieve and slip further into depression. The pain was trapped inside me with no way to surface. I continued to think about what I would leave behind. What would my obituary say? Somehow, wondering what would be said and be remembered about me suddenly became very important.

Being a stay-at-home mom, homemaker, cook, maid, etc, wasn't enough. At the end of the day, I had no accomplishments to list. I couldn't see that I was so blessed to be able to stay at home with my kids.

My life literally revolved around my kids. They controlled when I ate, slept, and took a shower. My baby had colic and cried constantly. Some nights I fell asleep on the hardwood floor, without a pillow or blanket, rubbing his arm while he sat in his bouncy chair. I wore pajamas every day because the effort to pick out real clothes was pointless. I wondered what had happened to the woman who wore suits, heels, and makeup.

The mixture of postpartum depression and the loss and grief for a loved one continued to pull me under. I felt trapped in a deep dark hole. I tried to pull free from the claws of depression, but every step I tried to take forward, ended up taking me further back. No one understood my feelings; I didn't even understand what was happening.

Everything seemed to take too much effort. I was sleep deprived, my body was trying to heal from the rigorous pregnancy and birth, and my heart was grieving. More than once, I wondered where God was and why did He leave me when I needed Him so much.

My life was not spanned in years or months, but days and sometimes just moments. My baby continued to develop more problems. He made odd noises when he breathed. We took multiple visits to the doctor and his long list of daily medications terrified me.

Every time I put the little mask over his face and gave him a breathing treatment, the realization that he needed the medicine to breath, slammed into me. Every time he rattled and wheezed, it terrified me. Every time I had sit for fifteen seconds and count his breaths while my heart pounded in my ears, I trembled with fear for the unknown. As the asthma attack increased in intensity and his breathing became more labored, he would plead with his eyes for me to help him.

At only a few months old, he took as many medications as most elderly people. They continued to run tests to try to determine the cause of his problems. When they mentioned cystic fibrosis, my heart dropped.

I walked the floors and prayed. In the middle of the night, while the world around me slept, I carried my precious baby many miles across the hardwood floors and wondered how long God would allow me to keep him. Even though all of the medical tests were negative and I was assured he only had asthma, allergies, and acid reflux, still watching him go through the effects of those conditions was heartbreaking. More than once, I wondered whether the doctors had missed something.

Finally, my extended maternity leave was over and it was time for me to return to work. How could I leave me sick child? I was so torn, but I knew I had to work to be able to afford his medicines and medical bills. My husband worked nightshift and I worked dayshift so our children wouldn't have to go to daycare.

There were pros and cons with our decision. One pro was that they would always have one of their parents with them, but that was also a con because that meant my husband and I were never there at the same time. After working all day, I had to come home and still do the same chores I had done while I was on maternity leave. There was no time for me, and I missed my kids so much.

I missed my husband, too. I cooked supper for the kids and I, then placed his plate in the refrigerator. I knew he would come home to a quiet house and feel as lonely as I felt, when he ate his supper alone.

Every day as I left for work, I thought about my life on the way. I wasn't content just being a stay-at-home mom, and I wasn't content working outside of my home and leaving my kids. I wished there were a way to find the best of both worlds.

I couldn't seem to focus on my work. My spirit was broken. I honestly didn't care what happened. The things that had once excited me and gave me a sense of accomplishment were gone and replaced with a sense of regret. I pulled away from my co-workers and slipped further into depression. Every morning when my eyes opened, I cringed at my long list of things that had to be done and prayed for the strength to keep going, because I was sure at any moment I would collapse into exhaustion.

One night there was restlessness inside me, as if I were missing something. I sat down on the couch, calmed myself, and listened for the voice of my Lord. Sometimes I would get a feeling like He wanted to talk to me. There was powerful feeling inside me to write. What? I didn't know. Instead of questioning the feeling, I complied.

In a blur of tears and words, coming so fast I could hardly keep up, a simple poem was recorded. I was shocked as I looked at the words blended together. All I could think as I read the poem again and again, was where did that come from? I was amazed! I, honestly, didn't know I could write something so beautiful. Now, I'm sure it wouldn't have impressed anyone else, especially, a publisher, but it was as if the grief welled up inside me for so long was gone - it was trapped on the paper instead of my heart.

I sat and held the poem for a long time and wondered what it meant. Careful not to wake the sleeping kids, I took my poem and retreated to the bathroom. It was a place where I thought and prayed. It was as if God compelled me to read it aloud. Unsure and shaky, I read the recorded words. My heart pounded, tears welled in my eyes. There was so much power in the words it terrified me. Then I heard my bedroom door slam and I cried, fearful that it would really be closed when I checked or even worse, that it would still be open. Curiosity pulled me from my safe haven and made me go see.

The door stood open just as I had left it, but the power still rushed through me. I knew it was God and He had something to tell me. I went back into the bathroom and looked at the very spot where I had kneeled years before and asked God to give me something that would be mine and some way to help others. As I held the poem in my hands, I knew God had just answered my prayer – He had opened a door for me.

Underneath the Scars

Chapter Three

The Diagnosis

And all things, whatsoever ye shall ask in prayer, believing, ye shall receive.
                                                                        -Matthew 21:22

Slowly, I began to climb out of the hole. Writing became my escape and my therapy. Whenever something overwhelmed me, I wrote about it. My son continued to have asthma attacks that terrified me, but recreating the scene later and putting it on paper, helped me to understand my feelings a little better.

Whatever happened to me, regardless of what the days held, somehow I knew I could escape it with words. Whenever I read the words written, it helped me to understand the person I was and the one I wanted to become. The person who held the pen wasn't afraid to reveal her emotions. My life felt more controlled and balanced. Instead of thinking about all of the things in my life that I couldn't control, I thought about the next story or poem I would write.

Nothing compared to the first poem, though. Occasionally, I would pull it out of my Bible and read it. Every time the simple words surfaced I remembered the power behind them and what I felt in my heart as I had written them. I remembered the college professor (in my only semester of college when I was eighteen) telling me to drop my law major and become an author. I had laughed then, but I wasn't laughing now. I remembered the young girl, who loved to write, but had been convinced it was foolish.

I wanted to continue further, yet it was as if something were holding me back. I believed in my heart that God had given me the gift to write, but questioned what He wanted me to pen. Every time the question surfaced, another question immediately formed in my mind: *What happened to my hands?*

It was like the elephant in the room. The quest to find my diagnosis plagued me. It wouldn't just go away. The question haunted me every day. I needed to know why I was chosen to bear the scars. But, all in the same sense, I was afraid to really know. It would change me (of that I was certain), but would it be a good or bad change? Was I strong enough to finally know the truth?

There was a reason for my scars and, in order to proceed with my life, I had to figure what had happened and perhaps even why. I knew God hadn't made a mistake. I didn't believe in the possibility of something just being a fluke of nature as others proclaimed. To me, that is like saying something slipped by God, beyond His control. I couldn't and wouldn't accept that possibility.

I didn't really know how to go about finding my diagnosis. In my twenty years plus, no doctor had ever been able to tell me anything. They always made me feel uncomfortable; it was as if they blamed me for what happened to my hands. They couldn't accept the fact that they didn't understand or have the diagnosis for my condition. Regardless of the reason for my visit, they always examined my hands and asked me several questions.

What happened to your hands? I don't know. I was just born this way.

Are there any other parts of your body affected? Yes, my foot and arm are affected too.

Did your mom take drugs? No!!!!

Was there an accident during pregnancy? No!

Is anyone else in your family affected? Nope, just me.

During their interrogation and examination, shame always slammed me in the face, even while my heart filled with hope. I endured the questions and examination of my scars because I hoped one day some doctor would finally diagnosis me. But each time they would make a comment about my scars being unusual and remaining an unsolved mystery.

In my heart, I knew the answers to my questions would come from God. Doctors can only take us so far. Even having extensive knowledge of the body doesn't mean they always know what happened or why. But God is all wise.

So I followed my heart. I sat down at the computer and began my search. I searched hand abnormalities, hand defects, and hand conditions. The amount of information that popped up was overwhelming. Since I had no clue what I was even searching for, I had to read everything. There were many big words I didn't understand, which meant I had to look them up as well.

And then I was faced with the problem, how would I know for certain that the condition I discovered was the same as mine?

Each time I sat down at the computer and began my search, I felt I was getting closer. Nevertheless, the nagging voice inside my head persisted that I didn't want to go down this road. What if I couldn't handle the truth? Was that the reason it had been shielded from me for so long? Would it change everything I was or everything I had known? Would it change the way I viewed myself entirely or how others viewed me?

In my heart, I knew the answers to my questions were YES!—but evening knowing that it *would* change me, I couldn't stop. I had to face my fears once and for all.

Apparently God believed it was time for me to learn the truth as well because the three little words that appeared in my search window beckoned for me to explore: *Amniotic Band Syndrome* (ABS).

My hands trembled as I clicked on the link. It wasn't just in the words, but the power I felt when I looked at those three words that had wreaked havoc on my life. Even if a million doctors told me it was some other condition, my heart knows it was indeed ABS.

Finally, the day I had dreamed about, wished for with my whole heart, and prayed for numerous times occurred. It appeared there was a diagnosis for my condition after all. There was a reason for my scars. Now, when someone asked me what happened to my hands, I would have an explanation. It would appease everyone's curiosity instead of my lifelong explanation of *I was born this way!*

I wanted to shout and sing and to call everyone I knew. I wanted to tell the world there was a purpose for my scars. I wanted to know everything there was to know about ABS.

The longer I searched, the more frustrated I became. The information was so vague and limited. It was technical and circumstantial. All I could find was a few pages at the most. After hours of researching, which turned into days, I was no closer to having my questions answered. If anything, I was more confused. Yes! I had a fancy name to associate with my scars, but that was it. When I stumbled onto the stories section of the website www.amnioticbandsyndrome.com and pictures of children affected, by the same condition, filled the screen - I was devastated.

Finding my diagnosis wasn't the magical occasion I had always anticipated. The tears that gushed down my face were not the tears of joy, I had always thought would accompany this day, but they were tears of sorrow. I thought I had already been through all of the trials and tribulations possible.

My initial reaction was shock. Somehow, I had believed, my whole life, I was the only person affected. To know there were others affected, too, didn't make me feel any better. If anything, it made my heart ache more to know there were other people who shared my world.

I took my time and clicked through the pictures of children missing limbs and digits. As the hot bitter tears raced down my cheeks, I touched the computer screen as if I could heal them. I wanted to take their scars away. I couldn't bear the thoughts of those beautiful smiling children facing the bitterness of life, I had so often encountered.

There were others forced to bear the stares and whispers I faced daily. There were others who would be judged unfairly throughout their life. There were others who would face the same trials and tribulations, I had faced. There were others who would cry themselves to sleep at night wishing their scars away. There were others who would struggle to find their own way of doing everything. There would be others plagued with the same fears that haunted me.

The air backed into my lungs. My mind raced. The silent tears turned into violent sobs. I grieved for the children affected as well as myself. I wanted to take them in my arms and tell them everything would be okay. I wanted to throw the best temper tantrum ever recorded history. Why was I so persistent on finding my diagnosis anyway? It wouldn't take away my scars. What would it change? Nothing! And then again – everything!

Why? Oh, God! Why?

I wanted and needed answers. With all of the advancements in modern medicine and billions of dollars spent in research each year, why couldn't anyone give me an explanation? Straight out, I wanted answers. I didn't want to hear, well maybe this happened or that happened. I wanted facts. I wanted solid evidence. Was it too much to ask for an explanation that was actually believable?

I couldn't continue reading the limited information. It was as if no one cared what had happened to cause ABS. No one had studied or researched it enough. There were no books or explanations.

Finally, exhausted and overwhelmed, I turned off the computer. I couldn't handle it. I was angry! Not only had God cursed me with scars, but also so many other children. I decided to forgo my continued research. Maybe I didn't want to know more about ABS after all. It was too heartbreaking.

The voice in my heart begged to differ. This wasn't the end, only the beginning.

Chapter Four

Answers to the Future Often Lie in the Past

And as Jesus passed by, he saw a man which was blind from his birth. And his disciples asked him, saying, Master, who did sin, this man, or his parents, that he was born blind? Jesus answered, Neither hath this man sinned, nor his parents: but that the works of God should be made manifest in him.

-John 9:1-3

I steered clear of the computer. It held images and words I didn't want to understand. Okay so I was being a coward, but I could live with that much better than I could live with the truth.

I tried to go on with my life even though it had been turned upside down. Regardless of where I was or what I was doing, images of children affected by ABS flashed before me. It was as if they beckoned me to help them. *What could I do?* I asked myself.

Words didn't comfort me. I lost the desire to write. There was too much inside me that I didn't want to deal with. I soon decided some things in life are better left buried. My quest to help others and to be an extraordinary person was too hard. I liked being ordinary and living a simple life, But oh wait, I wasn't ordinary either.

I quickly learned that you can't just forget something happened and go back to the life you lived before. This is going to sound insanely strange to you, I don't even understand it, but I felt cheated that there were others like me.

My whole life I had believed that I was the only one who had been born with these types of scars and to know there were others took away my uniqueness. It made me feel as if I had to suddenly compete with them, to constantly compare myself to them.

What if they had accomplished so much more in their life than I had? What if they had never whined and cried over their scars or dealt with fear? What if they had lived the life I had always dreamed of living?

Throughout this time, I learned another life lesson: courage is being terrified, but finding the strength to do it anyway. I could tell you that I found the strength inside myself to take the next step; however, in all reality, had God had not pushed me, I would still debating the issue and running from my feelings even today.

My next step was in an unlikely direction to the past. Talk about opening a whole new array of emotions. The only feelings I had had to deal with so far were my own feelings, and I wasn't prepared for what I encountered. My parents and I had never talked about my birth or any of the feelings associated with that day. I just assumed, because of their character, it was love at first sight. They had never made me feel as if I was anything less than my siblings. I was never the special child, the different child, the scarred child, nor anything less than simply Candida.

Some parents referred to their child's scars as their little arm, little hand, special hand, etc. and as I traveled in the past, I couldn't remember a time when my parents addressed my scars that way. They never said the hand with only one finger; it was simply my left hand. When they referred to my hands, there was no indication they saw my hands any different from my sibling's hands.

The gut-wrenching feeling that perhaps my parents had once had the same concerns broke my heart. They hadn't had support groups or even a diagnosis to explain my condition. How then did they get through it? How did they cope?

I began reliving my childhood in search of answers. I analyzed situations and how my parents acted toward me. I wondered if they had ever been ashamed of me. I drug out old photos and looked to see if my hands were hidden. And every picture was natural. If my hands were visible they were photographed. To appease my curiosity, I asked my mom about the day I was born. I expected her to give me some beautiful story and tell me it had never been an issue, but it once was devastating to them.

I sat in silence as my mom relieved the day I was born. Silent tears fell as I listened to her story.

It was a day filled with anticipation, pink lacey dresses, and the hope of a healthy child. The nursery was prepared with new clothes, lotions, toys, and anything else imaginable that a newborn might need. They only thing still needed was the baby.

My parents wanted a little girl. My name had been selected and my future decided. They had it all planned out: how they would juggle the financial cost, my pediatrician, middle of the night feedings, diapers, etc. Already the parents of a four-year-old boy, they weren't blind to the demands of a baby. They had been through pregnancy, labor, delivery, the heartaches and joys of raising a child, previously. They knew what to expect!

Underneath the Scars

The delivery was routine as well as the pregnancy, and never through it all, did anyone expect the outcome. It wasn't until the first wail burst from my lungs, accompanied by the weary expression on the doctor's face, that my parents realized something was wrong. The doctor was a professional, with hundreds of babies delivered, yet had never seen a child look like the one he was holding.

Their normalcy was shattered. In an attempt to comfort my parents and hopefully lessen their shock, the doctor rushed me away without allowing them one simple glance or an explanation. The loving arms, which waited for many months were empty. Their miraculous day turned tragic. As imaginations soared and grief consumed them, all they had to hold onto was hope, prayers, and love.

Despite the medical training provided and the initials after his name, the physician could not offer a diagnosis or prognosis. What was he to tell the parents who were expecting and hoping for a perfect child? How was he to explain what had happened, when he had no clue himself? There was neither rhyme nor reason; just a child with scars and questions with no answers.

The best he could offer was a description, to hopefully lessen the shock and prepare them for what they would soon face. My left hand had only the pinkie finger; the other four fingers were joined together by bone, joints, and nerves. The hand resembled a mitten. All four fingers appeared to be amputated after the first knuckle and nothing more than a stub. On the right hand, all of the fingers were joined and just barely past the second knuckle. None of the fingers were formed normally. Some type of unknown band had wrapped around my right arm near the bicep and had left an impression. The left foot had the big toe joined with second toe, and the remaining toes didn't match the other foot.

The happiness anticipated for months turned to heartache, bitterness, and anger! Why? How? It had to be a horrible nightmare. It couldn't be real. There had to be an explanation. While some thought it was nothing more than a fluke of nature, others wondered why God would do that to a child. What had my parents done to cause me to be born that way? Where there drugs involved? Was it caused by a vitamin deficiency? Was it genetic?

With thousands of questions speculated, rumors gossiped, pity offered, and prayers prayed, my mom lay in her bed and wondered what she had done to cause my scars. Even though she knew in her heart that she hadn't done anything wrong, still the blame overcame her already broken heart. She relived the pregnancy over and over, searching for answers.

All of their hopes and dreams for my future shattered like a fine vase. My parents weren't ready for a special child with special needs.

Finally, overwhelmed with emotions and fears, my mom sent for me. The nurse brought me bound in a blanket with my scars hidden. Even with a description, my mom was terrified to remove the covering. She snuggled me, caressed my face, kissed me, and apologized. She tried to find the courage to reveal my hands, but the fear prevailed. She prayed it was only a misunderstanding; that under the blankets, my hands were perfect and there were no scars. She held me tight, afraid to look, wishing for strength and comfort.

And then, God intervened.

Underneath the Scars

I removed my hands, bound by the blanket, and laid them on her face. In all reality, it was impossible, but with God all things are possible. He opened her heart to me. In that moment, she fell in love. She didn't know how it would all work, but she knew God would help us. I wasn't handicapped or defective as some claimed - I was a miracle from God.

Tears poured down the faces of family members and friends as they heard the news and circumstances of my birth. However, not everyone viewed me as a miracle. To some I would always be defected, to others definitely handicapped and different with no chance of a normal life. I would never be independent, never be beautiful, never play the piano, or do all of the things normal people do. I would always be a burden; my parents would have to find the strength to care for me.

While my fate was being decided, I had no idea that I was different. I acted as any other baby, with perhaps an extra boost of determination.

My parents knew I was not a typical child, but they never dreamed I would grow up and be so independent or stubborn. I insisted on feeding myself, even once with my arm in a sling. I crawled, walked, and in all reality, acted as all other children. I found a way (my own way) to do everything. I didn't require therapy or any special assistance to do anything. I was on the same level with my peers, and if anything, I was more advanced.

My parents loved me tremendously and even seeing all of the accomplishments I had made, they still clung to the hope that a plastic surgeon could repair the damage, not because they were vain, but because they wanted the best for me. They never wanted me to hurt or to struggle in life.

Because there were no local doctors available with any knowledge of a hand abnormality, a hand surgeon came from afar to evaluate me. My parents' hopes were crushed again. The nerves entwined in my hands made surgery an unlikely option. The odds were stacked unfavorably. If he attempted to separate the joined fingers, one wrong move could completely destroy any functionality, and no amount of plastic surgery could improve the appearance.

In addition, regardless of the medical knowledge and advancements, the specialist could not provide a diagnosis or answer their questions. But he did offer a prognosis. "God gave her to you this way and if you try to change her He might take her. She will be gifted in some way and one day you will see it. Take her home, love her, and always encourage and support her," he told them.

When my mom finished the story of my birth, I wondered why my mom had never shared it before. Although there were parts of my story that were hard to hear, I wanted to give my parents a standing ovation. Knowing they had struggled with my birth, but still managed to raise me the way they had, made my respect for them so much greater.

I edged further and talked to my siblings. While growing up, I was sure they were ashamed me, but I was told they looked up to me and respected me. They always believed in me and loved me. Their faith and adoration overwhelmed me.

It both amazes and aggravates me at how people view others. For my whole life, it has been assumed that my parents were burdened with me because of some sin they committed. I thought about the gift the hand surgeon spoke about, and in my heart, I knew that was what God had planned for me all along.

Chapter Five

Learning to Overcome Obstacles

But Jesus beheld them, and said unto them, With men this is impossible; but with God all things are possible.
-Matthew 19:26

I wasn't sure I knew or understood the person I was, anymore. So many emotions I thought I had overcome (or at least dealt with) were pounding on the dam of my heart. Already my vision of my birth had been altered. What was next? Was everything about my life different? I felt as if I were standing back looking in, and it was someone else's life I was viewing.

My mom and I began to talk more about my childhood. There was a great need inside of me to know everything. I had to face all of the demons in my closet. And let me assure you, it was not an easy thing to do.

Throughout this process, many times I thought that what we don't know can't hurt us. But it *was* hurting me. I needed to lay all of the cards on the table and deal with each situation.

Having children of my own gave me an advantage. I thought about all of the things I worried about with my own children and then asked my mom about those things in my own life. Because school was an issue for everyone, I started there.

Underneath the Scars

Kindergarten: it's the dreaded day all parents despise. The baby that once cooed, drooled, and toddled has become a kindergartener and the apron strings are getting shorter and shorter.

I remember how I felt the first day I took my little boy to school and dropped him off. I worried his new shoes would hurt his feet, he would forget his backpack, he would feel alone and left out, he wouldn't be able to open his milk carton, and no one would play with him or sit with him at lunch. Who would wipe his nose, button his pants, or lay with him at naptime? Despite all of my worries, I can't even begin to imagine how my mom felt leaving me alone in a school with so many silent questions and magnetic stares. For the first time in my life, her body couldn't shield me from the gawking that happened daily, without me noticing. She couldn't reroute a stare with a smile or stern glare, nor offer an explanation when someone made a rude comment. She was forced to walk away and leave me alone and vulnerable.

As bad as that sounds, I was never truly alone. Prayers comforted me and God shielded me from the cruel reality of life. I am sure the kids gaped at me and perhaps even the staff at the school, but if I noticed, I don't remember. I think the biggest reason is because I wasn't expecting them to stare at me. I had never been subject to that kind of behavior, so I didn't constantly expect it to happen.

I was, however, very shy. Regardless of the times my parents praised me, or told me I was beautiful, their opinion didn't really matter because I expected them to say those things. What mattered was how my peers viewed me. I wanted them to like me. And because I feared they wouldn't, I became timid. I don't really know whether my feelings had anything to do with my scars or whether it was simply because I didn't know anyone. I had never been in a position in which I had to make friends on my own. Previously, I had played with other kids at church and birthday parties, or with cousins who visited our house with their parents. Making friends at school was different, though. I can remember standing by myself, watching all of the other kids play and being afraid to approach them and ask whether I could play too.

Kindergarten was a frustrating time for me as well as my teacher. Not only was I upset because I wanted to stay home with my mom and baby sister, but also was a girl born with obstacles in her way. Each day was trial and error.

It was difficult for someone with ten fingers to instruct someone with only five – both hands combined – to do a simple task. To be honest, when people see you struggle to complete tasks, they assume you're disabled or handicapped. It was my opportunity to show the world I was neither.

My mom had one request for the school. They were told to treat me as they did the other children. No special treatment! She didn't ask the school to adapt to me, but she forced me to adapt to it. There were no special scissors, crayons, or pencils. I used the same supplies as children with five fingers on each hand. I was given the same amount of time to complete my work as my peers. I didn't have a special aid to assist me or even someone to help me figure out how to make my hands do the things that needed to be done.

For the most part, everything came natural. I just picked up my pencil, held it in my hand where it was comfortable, and wrote. Scissors, on the other hand, became a definite trial. My index finger was attached to my middle and ring finger, so in order to use scissors, I had to hold those three fingers up or curve them and use my short thumb and curved pinky finger; which made using scissors difficult, but not impossible (they're still rather challenging at times).

Everything worked for a while, but then one day I came home crushed. Every child in my class got to paint their handprints for their parents except for me. The next day my mom marched into the school and demanded answers. Why wasn't I allowed to do handprints? When she found out it was because the teacher didn't think she would want them, my mom was furious. By the time she left, everyone at the school understood my hands were as special to her as any other child's hands were to their parents. Needless to say, I did my handprints.

Some are so uncomfortable around people who are different that they offend them unintentionally. Perhaps my teacher thought it would have hurt my mom to see my handprints. I don't believe she intentionally tried to hurt my mom or me. Even through a blanket of tears, the whole experience helped me in the long run. It forced the faculty at the school to look at me as they did the other children, or at least try to understand that my mom wanted me to have a regular life.

That was a defining moment in my life! Even though I don't remember all the details, it was a stepping-stone toward an ordinary life for me.

If you want people to treat you normal, you act normal, right? If my mom had waltzed into the school with a long list of demands and instructions, would anyone have ever treated me normal? No! If I were always the child with special equipment, then, yes, I would be 'the special child' to everyone. And I don't mean that in a good way.

Perhaps schools are forced to adapt to the special needs of their students, but I assure you the world doesn't adapt for anyone. Not to mention, very few employers would consider hiring an employee that needed special supplies and equipment, or who expected special treatment.

Now that you're steaming and seriously getting mad at me, please let me clarify a bit. There are those seriously affected that do require special treatment and special equipment. For example, someone paralyzed needs a wheelchair to maneuver, but they don't need someone to constantly do everything for them out of pity. Yes, they will work harder than most to complete the same tasks, but regardless they can and will do it. Sometimes it only requires minor adjustments to make things easier. And sometimes we learn to do things even though to an outsider it looks impossible. My hands are all I've ever known. So, of course, I can use them and make them do whatever needs to be done. Just because I can't pick up a glass the way someone else does, doesn't mean I can't pick it up. Nor does it mean I need some extra assistance. In all reality, all I need is for people to understand. It may take me a while to figure out how to make my one finger on my left hand, do what your five fingers can do, but I can and will.

When I was in elementary school, sports were hard for me, especially baseball. I always dreaded batting. The force of the ball hitting the bat hurt my hands tremendously. Regardless of how I tried to hold the bat, still the connection made me wince and left my hands throbbing. Perhaps I should have told my teacher in the beginning, but I didn't want anyone to look at me as though I were handicapped, so I tried to deal with it the best I could. Fielding was also hard. The gloves didn't fit my hands, and it made it hard for me to catch the ball in the gloved hand because even if it hit my hand, I couldn't keep it there. Finally, I couldn't take the aggravation of playing baseball any longer and I mentioned it to my P.E. teacher. Instead of understanding my limitations, he told an inspirational story to the whole class. It didn't make me feel better to know that a certain baseball player with similar limitations mastered the craft. I felt singled out, and everyone in my class knew the story was targeted toward me. I felt ashamed that I couldn't play baseball, a simple thing that every child should be able to do.

Looking back at that whole incident now, I understand more about why I couldn't play baseball. There was no passion. With a little love of the sport, I would have worked harder trying to find a way around my limitations. But as it were, the effort to learn was far greater than the reward of playing. We all have to choose our battles in life. No one is great at everything. The things we are truly passionate about, we strive to do our best. All others are cast aside.

I do believe I can do ANYTHING that I truly want to do, but there has to be a greater force driving me than the one trying to stop me.

In high school, I decided to take driver's education because it would reduce my insurance premiums, and it was the thing to do. I was excited about the class, and always respected the teacher. However, when I became his student, things changed. He automatically assumed, based on the appearance of my hands, that I couldn't drive. I was discriminated from the first day. I'll admit I couldn't drive very well, but once again it had nothing to do with my hands and everything to do with lack of experience and practice.

Instead of looking at the whole class and the percentage of students who were in my range, it was just easier to treat me as if I were handicapped. The teacher made a huge issue out of my hands and even fixed the steering wheel with cardboard because, in his opinion, that would make it easier for me to grip. Despite the humiliation, I refused to give up and drop his class. On one hand, it pushed me harder and I was determined to get my driver's license; while on the other hand, it caused doubt to flicker in my mind. What if the instructor of the driver's license office discriminated against me as well? Those doubts and fears clung to me daily. If I failed my driving test and never got my license then I would always be dependent on others. And that fear was what made me go to my parents for help.

Once again, my mom went to school and demanded they treat me as any other student. The principal, obviously troubled over the issue, called the State of Kentucky to inquire whether I would be permitted to continue the class. When he told them on the phone I had a hand disability, I nearly jumped out of my chair. Never, in the three years I had attended the school, did I once ever ask for special treatment or assistance in any class. I took and passed all of the required courses. Nevertheless, because one teacher only saw scars when he looked at me, I was labeled as disabled. Needless to say, after the intervention, I got to continue with my driver's education, but the thrill and excitement of learning to drive was taken away from me. It became a burden.

Even some members of family thought driving was something I would never accomplish. Instead of listening to all of the doubts (because I had enough of my own), I listened to my heart. I knew that even if I failed and never learned to drive it wouldn't be for a lack of trying. It was one of those times in life when we are tested. I felt as if the whole world were watching and waiting to see what happened. I knew if I failed my test and never got my license that even the possibility of a normal life would be shattered. The thought that everyone – even the people who believed I was special – would look at me differently and be forced to see me as handicapped terrified me and made me try harder.

My dad, with great patience and understanding, worked with me. And, even though I've never asked, I'm sure there were prayers prayed for me too. If truth be known, my daddy probably prayed the whole time I was driving, because I scared him to death. However, he NEVER gave up on me, nor allowed me to give up on myself. The first time I took my driving test, I was so nervous. My fears overpowered me and I failed. It happened; the worst possible scenario and yet I survived. I was devastated and more determined than ever before. I REFUSED to give up. I continued practicing and the next time I took my test, I was confident and I passed. I learned to drive because I wanted it so badly. I didn't give up because it was something that was just too hard. I practiced until I finally succeeded. And the feeling of success definitely overpowered the heartache.

I realized after my journey through time to my school days that things have always been hard for me, but I've always been able to overcome any obstacle in my way. We all have physical as well as mental strengths and weaknesses. But when we learn to combine our strengths with our weaknesses is when we find success. All of the struggles I faced during my quest to get my driver's license made the victory so much sweeter. It showed me anything is possible if we want it badly enough.

Chapter Six

Heartaches and Fears

And now, Israel, what doth the LORD thy God require of thee, but to fear the LORD thy God, to walk in all his ways, and to love him, and to serve the LORD thy God with all thy heart and with all thy soul.
                                                               -Deuteronomy 10:12

Traveling back in time to my own experiences made my heart heavier for the children with ABS and my desire to help them even stronger. Reliving the past, through memories, made me realize the worst part of living with ABS was not the actual trials and tribulations, but the fears and what ifs.

Since the information about ABS is so limited and I didn't have a name for my condition when I was growing up, the fear of the unknown slammed me daily. In my experience, the horror of something happening is always worse than when it actually happens – if it even does, that is. Nevertheless, we always tend to believe the worst and that we are not strong enough to handle certain situations.

I never wanted to write about my fears; they just seem too personal to share with others. I've come to understand, though, that sometimes by sharing our own experiences we help others.

As far back as I can remember, fear has overwhelmed me. I can remember staring in the mirror trying to figure out who I was and what was my purpose in life. Some people referred to me as a special child. I asked myself, *What's so special about me?* Since when did freckles, red hair, and scars warrant the title of special? I didn't have any magical powers (even though I tested my hands a few times). I couldn't climb walls, shoot anything, or make my hands do anything neat. There were just there, broken and scarred.

Fear plagued me, every time I picked something up, every time a new task emerged, every time someone stared at me, and every time I looked at my scars.

There were so many nights my tears lulled me to sleep; when the pressure of it all seemed too much. I wanted to escape the horrible nightmare that appeared into reality. I wanted it to be a dream that the morning light would chase away. But every day I was reminded, before I even opened my eyes, I couldn't escape.

It was a fearful thing to stand before a world that demanded perfection. Exposed and afraid, I faced stares and whispers daily. The first time someone's eyes darted to my hands broke my heart. But worse than that was the pity that usually flashed in their eyes before they looked away. All they could see was a girl with two broken wings trying to survive. Some respected my determination, while others were pessimistic that I would ever amount to anything. Honestly, I think the doubt splattered on those faces helped me to persevere.

The older I got, the harder my fears were to manage. I was more aware of the stares and whispers. I realized when people were indeed laughing at me, instead of laughing with me. I noticed when I was excluded and how others viewed me. People think they can be smooth and cover their shock or rudeness, but their true feelings are in their eyes. Regardless of what they say, their eyes tell the whole story.

Of course they could smile and tell me how beautiful I was, but when their eyes drifted to my scars and looked repulsed, I knew how they really felt about me. That was the one of hardest parts for me; the unspoken words.

When I entered into the teenage years, I felt so alone. People weren't as kind to me as they had been when I was a child. It was an unknown world and I wasn't sure how to survive. As much as I wanted to crawl into my parent's arms and allow their comfort to surround me, another part wanted to prove I could handle it. I wanted my independence

I wanted to go on dates and flirt with boys like my peers, but I was shy and terribly self-conscious. Instead of being outgoing and fun, I tried to blend in with my surroundings and hide my scars. I shoved my hands in my pockets as often as I could, hoping people would forget.

I longed to be someone's best friend and I wished, just once, someone could look at me and think I was beautiful. I had a picture hanging on my wall of a little girl that read, "The only way to have a friend is to be one."

And I tried so hard to be a good friend, but many times I was too afraid to be the real me. So often, I was frightened to stand for what I believed in or voice my opinion because I didn't want to give anyone another reason to dislike me. I was also easily influenced because the desire to be included was so fierce. I went with the crowd whether it was right or wrong. I stood in the shadows, while everyone else lived, because the fear of rejection terrified me.

Underneath the Scars

    I learned to not expect much out of life, I failed to see the bright side of anything. I decided to expect the worse and that way when it happened, the disappointment wouldn't be as tough. I went through the motions of life. My smiles were forced and my laughter was a foreign sound that I no longer heard. For a good while, I wallowed in self-doubt lathered with pity and tried to give up. Life was not easy for me. Constantly, I was asked to prove myself, and honestly, I got tired of being looked at underneath a microscope.

    Every evening, after school, I crawled into my bed and dreamed of the life I wanted, but could never have. I dreamed of the prom dress I would never wear. In my mind, I knew exactly the shape, texture, and color, yet I could never (not even in my dreams) see myself wearing it. It was as if I were standing behind the glass of life and couldn't make my way into reality. Eventually, I pulled away from family. In my mind, I had failed them and myself.

    I was afraid I would never find a partner to love me and see past my imperfections into my heart. But you see I didn't just want love, I wanted the fairy tale love like my parents and grandparents shared, and I refused to settle for anything less than what I thought I deserved. I wanted the whole package, the knight in shining armor, who would sweep me off my feet and leave me ruined for every other man. I had big dreams and even bigger expectations. But how could I expect anyone to ask me for forever, when I would ask them to love me the way I am?

    Living with the unknown was especially difficult. I had a zillion questions and no one could answer them (and I didn't ask the one who could!). I was terrified one day my hands would refuse to work and I would be the handicapped girl, everyone perceived me to be. The thought of relying on others to care me and for my survival overwhelmed me. I couldn't imagine watching life happen around me without being able to participate. There were so many things I still had to face; either to conquer or fail.

A life without the pitter-patter of little feet, sticky kisses, and unexpected hugs was an unbearable thought. From the moment I changed a pretend diaper for my baby Sara I knew, one day, I wanted to be a real mom. A part of me thought wanting to have children was selfish. Since there was no diagnosis for my condition how could I (or anyone else for that matter) be sure my condition wasn't genetic? How could I ever look at my child bearing my scars and not be ashamed I caused their grief? How could I ask another soul to bear my heartaches?

Each fraction of rejection and failure pushed me closer to my fears and soon they multiplied. I focused more on the things I couldn't do, rather than all the things I could do

I allowed my fears to dwell in the depth of my heart. I lived for the future rather than the present. The 'what ifs' of life nearly drove me crazy. An imagination can be a wonderful thing, but it can also be the devil in disguise.

My biggest mistake was not turning my burdens over to God. I thought I was strong enough to handle it all, and in turn created more problems. Looking back now I wished I had asked God for the strength to accept myself, verses asking God to heal my hands.

As much as I wanted to stay in my bed with the covers pulled over my head, the desire to live instead of merely existing overwhelmed me. I wanted to be happy!

Underneath the Scars

    The first step was realizing no one could make me happy and that I deserved to be! It was a choice I had to make for myself. I made bad decisions, some I still regret, but I learned so many lessons from my mistakes. One of the greatest things I learned was to be me, regardless of the repercussions.

    During my, what if my world felt apart crisis, I didn't realize I was judging other people unfairly. I didn't believe they could look past the exterior and see me. I assumed all of these bad things without any of them actually happening. I didn't have enough faith in God, myself, or others. Finally, I realized the fear of falling down was worse than actually falling down and I would never know until I tried.

Chapter Seven

Blinded by Scars

He will deliver his soul from going into the pit, and his life shall see the light.
-Job 33:28

    The summer I turned seventeen, the school offered a program for low-income families. It was an opportunity for me to get a job. Transportation was provided and I qualified based on my family's financial situation. Although some looked down their nose at a job like that, I saw it as a golden opportunity. It was a chance for me to prove I could work. And the wages earned would buy me new school clothes and the emerald green contacts I desperately wanted.

    However, the paycheck I earned every two weeks wasn't the only reward I received.

    My fears accompanied me my first day. I wasn't sure how my co-workers would feel working with me. How would they treat me? Would they stare at me? My unanswered questions almost paralyzed me and had me wanting to give up before I even tried. In my heart, I knew not trying would be much worse than failing. So I pushed my fears aside and walked in with a smile on my face, trembling knees, and a stomach full of butterflies.

Underneath the Scars

I was greeted with friendly smiles and loving hearts. The job was exciting. I was a receptionist. Each new task I learned and eventually mastered, provided confidence; something I was really lacking. I loved working with adults. They treated me differently than my peers had. I loved the responsibility and sense of accomplishment each workday provided. Even though I was only seventeen, I felt much older. I matured during that summer and realized I wanted to live. I was tired of only existing.

I was a different person when the job ended than when it began. I took my money and bought new clothes to go with my new attitude. And the only thing still lacking was my contacts. I made my appointment and walked in unaware of the challenges awaiting me.

Because I didn't really need contacts, the doctor pacified me and gave me the weakest ones available. I picked out the vibrant color and was thrilled to wear them. And that's where the challenge emerged. I couldn't put them in with my hands. I was devastated. I wanted to cry and storm out; determination stopped me. If I gave up every time something was hard for me then I would never succeed in life. I listened as the assistant suggested I get glasses instead. I didn't want glasses—I wanted contacts; emerald green contacts to be exact. I assured her I would, eventually, master it. She must have seen a flicker of my determination because she agreed. I can't remember whether she put them in for me or whether I did it myself, but I left with contacts in my eyes.

I was determined to put my contacts in every day. Granted I had to get up for school an hour earlier to do a simple task most people complete in a few minutes; nevertheless, I eventually learned my own way.

Working had ruined me. I wasn't content not having a job. However, this time it would be different. I would have to prove that I *deserved* the job. I would have to go through the application and interview process, and it terrified me. How would I convince anyone I was qualified for a job when the job required ten fingers and I only had half that amount (both hands combined)? What did I possibly have to offer any employer than someone else couldn't offer?

During an interview for a waitressing position, the manager asked me if I thought I could do it. I told him I honestly didn't know, but I wanted the opportunity to try, and in the event I failed, I would admit my defeat and quit. The answer seemed to satisfy him because I started immediately.

For the first time in my life, my parents, friends, and entire family didn't believe in me. No one thought I could waitress. And to be honest I wasn't entirely sure myself. But I refused to accept failure based on fear and lack of trying.

Once again, I was submerged into a place where everyone did things differently. And I was afraid. Standing ALONE in the middle of that restaurant was a defining moment in my life. In the depths of my heart, I hoped I could do it.

The possibility that I would fail was always in the back of my mind. The first time I put on my uniform and picked up my tray, I knew I had risked everything. If I wasn't able to do it all of my friends and family would know I had failed. While some might give me credit for trying, for the most part, sympathy would be offered. I couldn't bear the thought of everyone knowing I couldn't do a simple job. I couldn't bear the thought of my hands proving, I was in fact handicapped.

The victory didn't come easy or without hardships. I couldn't carry the trays like other waitresses. I couldn't carry as many pitchers, or hold the glasses as they did. At first, it was so frustrating for me. I had to make extra trips from the waitressing station to the dining room, but still received the same pay. I believed, with years of experience in finding my own way, it was possible to do the job as good as my co-workers. My left hand was weak from years of favoring my right hand, but in order to improve I knew I had to strengthen my left hand.

It was hard, and at times it started throbbing before half my shift was completed, but I gritted my teeth and continued to push myself. Defeat was a word I didn't intend to use. Before I knew it, I had developed strategies to help me make my trips back and forth more productive.

I was treated as an equal to the other servers. I was never given less tables or an easier section. Toward the end, I even requested the busiest sections. And there were a few times, when I covered the whole dining room myself. To be honest, I think people didn't always realize I was different. I never mentioned my hands. I didn't walk up to the tables and make excuses for myself.

I've often thought about that job. Sympathy might have gotten me the job, but hard work and determination enabled me to keep it. Of all the jobs I've ever had, that one holds a special place in my heart. It constantly challenged me to push myself to the limit and I amazed myself on many occasions. It gave me confidence. It was a job that required ten fingers and still I found a way to do it.

Comments were made by rude, pessimistic people who claimed I only received tips out of pity or sympathy, but in my heart I begged to differ. I did the job that I was paid to do, and all the tips I collected were deserved and appreciated.

All too soon, I realized that not every employer shared the same goodwill. While most businesses have a pretty sign claiming they are an equal opportunity employer, are they really?

No!

People can say what they want, and perhaps some even believe they are totally fair, but until you've been looked upon as being handicapped, you wouldn't understand. It is all in the eyes, they never lie. A fake smile, while trying to swallow the gasp of shock, is obvious, regardless of how well they try to cover it up.

One of the hardest blows of my life came when I was just eighteen years old. I worked as a cashier in a country store, in my hometown, while I went to college. My employer was a woman I had known my whole life. She knew my story. She was a friend of the family, someone I went to church with, and someone I respected. There were people who tried to warn me about her because they believed she would hurt me, but I had faith in her. I never thought for one minute she would hurt me. Regardless of all the bad things people said about her, I saw the good in her.

I worked for her for a few weeks, maybe a month, before I was taken off the schedule. When I inquired why, she told me we needed to talk before I returned to work.

I must give her credit she didn't dance around the issue; she got straight to the point. I was fired that day because I couldn't wring out a mop good enough. Point blank, she fired me because of my hands and she didn't try to hide it. She said I was also too slow and made some of the customers feel awkward.

I'm sure I've been hurt worse in my life, but that was a low blow. I was ashamed! I was so hurt! I was a failure! My education, struggles to succeed, and ambitions were pointless. All of my accomplishments were forgotten. It wasn't about all I had overcome and learned to do, it all came down to the one thing I couldn't do.

It was a horrible misunderstanding. That's what I wanted to believe. I expected her to call me and tell me she was wrong. That she hadn't meant all of the horrible things she had said to me. With every day I became more blinded by the anger and hurt.

I grieved and tried to give up. What was I fighting for anyway? If the world was going to look at me as being handicapped and stand in my way when I tried to make something of myself, then why even bother? I was ashamed when I went out into the public. I felt as if everyone was condemning me. And the pity accompanying their expressions broke my heart. I didn't want pity. My hopes of living a normal life vanished.

I wallowed in self-pity for a while. I didn't even try to get back up. I was comfortably knocked down and, to be honest, I wanted to stay down. It was easier to accept my failure and just not try. If I were going to be treated like I was handicapped, then I would act like it.

And then I thought about it. I would have no life. No purpose. I would sit at home with little or no friends and feel sorry for myself every second of every day. There would be no goals, no ambitions, no success, and very little happiness. Every day would be a failure. I would disappoint God (not to mention myself). While there are a few things I can't do, my ability surpasses any disability. God would be disappointed not because of the few things I couldn't do, but of all the things I refused to do because I was scared.

Even though I know we are not supposed to question God, I found myself doing just that. Why would God allow anyone to hurt me so deeply? I tried to pray, but the anger stood in my way. I wallowed in it for a while, vowing I would NEVER forgive and forget. I would hate and be proud of myself for doing it. After all, I had a good reason for hating her, didn't I?

As much as I wanted to justify my feelings, there was no excuse or reason I could fine that allowed me to hate anyone.

Blinded by the scars in my heart, I took some time to realize that I had to forgive in order to move on. And even though, eventually, I wanted to forgive and forget; it wasn't that easy. My question was how do you forgive someone that is not even sorry they hurt you? She continued to live her life as if nothing had ever happened, while I was miserable.

I wanted revenge. I wanted her to hurt, just as I had. Or at least that's what I told myself. When I searched my heart, I realized she hurt me so deeply because I loved her, respected her, and admired her. Not only had I lost my job, but I had lost our friendship. I wished over and over the whole incident had never happened. I wanted her to hug me and apologize.

Then, I thought about Jesus. While He was hanging on the cross for our sins, He didn't lash out with vengeance. He could have come off that cross at any time, but love for us held Jesus there. He died for the ones who had beaten and mocked Him, just as he did you and me. He loved even ones who hated Him.

I didn't get it the first few times I tried, but I did eventually find the strength to forgive, totally and completely. I buried all of my hard feelings and replaced them with love. Regardless of how she felt about me – I loved her. I was very sorry the whole incident happened, but I refused to dwell on it any longer.

There is nothing anyone can do to change the past. I realized I had to move forward. I didn't want to be a bitter person or someone who held a grudge. I refused to be blinded by my hurts and didn't want anything or anyone to stand in my way of serving God. Nothing is more important that God! And let's be honest, can anyone serve God while hating their brother? No! God is love!

Once I reached forgiveness and put the situation behind me, I was able to move forward. As much as I wanted to jump back up and pretend I was the same person, prior to what happened, I knew that I wasn't. Wanting to get up was the first step, and asking God to help me was the most important.

Even though I had moved on, I was still a little gun-shy. Although I was terrified it would happen again, I began applying for new jobs.

The first day I put in applications, I got a job before I even made it back home. It wasn't a fascinating job, but a job nevertheless. This time I had something to prove to myself. Once I mastered all of the duties and performed as well as any other employee, my confidence increased.

God didn't prevent me from being hurt, but He did strengthen me because of it. One of my biggest fears in life had happened and I survived it. I got back up! The love that dwells in my heart helped me to prevail!

The whole incident opened my blinded eyes and taught me a lesson. Some breeze through life while others struggle, and so often, the difficult times are what mold us. In life, when things don't go the way we intended, we have two choices: we can either turn away from God, blaming Him for our troubles, or we can turn into His strong, comforting arms and lay our head on His shoulder as He carries us.

Today, believe it or not, I look at this whole incident as a blessing. Yes! Bad things will happen to me in my life. I will hurt. I will doubt myself, occasionally. There'll be times when everything seems so hopeless, but God is always there. There is NOTHING that can or will happen to me that God won't help me overcome. There is no pain or disappointment so great that God can't comfort me.

People will always try to hurt us, but they can only really hurt us if we allow them to. I've learned anytime we can take our anger and turn it into tears, love conquers. I've learned to pray for those who hurt me. As a little girl, I was always taught to shower them with kindness. Think about it, how would you feel if the person you were mean to was on their knees praying for you? Real strength is not fighting back with cruelty when people hurt you, but fighting back with love. Love can defeat the strongest enemy, every single time.

I saw the light.

Underneath the Scars

And we know that all things work together for good to them that love God, to them who are the called according to his purpose.
-Romans 8:28

Chapter Eight

Confidence is Earned

He giveth power to the faint; and to them that have no might he increaseth strength.
-Isaiah 40:29

In some ways with my first jobs, I had proved that I wasn't handicapped (even though one employer begged to differ). I had waitressed, cashiered, and retailed, yet at the end of every day I felt I still had something more to prove. I wanted a job that pushed me harder and further than I had ever been before. I needed to excel.

I was very timid during interviews because the minute my hands were addressed I closed up. I didn't have the courage to look anyone in the eye and tell them I wasn't handicapped when the doubt flickered every once in a while. I realized that if I wanted a job worth anything, I would have to overcome my insecurities.

The first time I was interviewed for a clerical position, I was required to take a typing test. My hands shook and my legs trembled. For the first time in my life, my hands would be tested and the basis for whether or not I got the job. My anxiety bubbled, and I'm sure, fear danced in my eyes. I wanted to refuse and run, but stubbornness made me sit in the chair and at least try.

The keyboard felt foreign. Half way through, I wanted to quit. The fear of failure overwhelmed me. I was intimidated. I knew before the test was graded that I had failed miserably. The interview following the exam was even worse. The pity on her face haunted me. She was polite and just talked to me about my hands. The potential job was never discussed.

I kept a smile on my face until I left – even though I wanted to tell everyone where to go and how to get there. The moment I walked outside, the restrained tears fell like a raging waterfall, and I grieved.

I refused to accept defeat. I realized that if I wanted to work as a secretary or other clerical position, then I needed to learn to type. However, there were no books or instruction manuals to teach my hands how to move. It would take patience, determination, and lots of practice.

Every time I felt like giving up, I recalled that particular interview and refused to ever repeat that type of insult again. Not only did I need to learn and master the skills, but I also needed confidence.

I polished my resume until is shined. Then, I practiced in the mirror. I pulled my shoulders back, held my head up, and told my reflection over and over I wasn't handicapped. I practiced listing my pitiful qualifications, and the reasons I wanted the job, until I convinced myself.

When the next interview occurred, I was ready. I dressed in my best suit and spent extra time on my appearance. That gave me an extra boost of confidence. While I wasn't sure whether I would get the job or not, I was determined not to let anyone play the handicapped card. If I didn't get the job, it would be because I was not qualified, not because the potential employer decided I was handicapped.

I entered the interview confidently and with a smile on my face. I shook his hand and made eye contact. After all, I had nothing to be ashamed of. I answered his questions and listened as he explained the job's duties. It seemed like a dream job to me. I wanted it so bad.

When he addressed my hands, for a moment, I hesitated. Then I thought what do I have to lose? I smiled at him and assured him I was not handicapped. Courage surrounded me and I guaranteed him with the proper training I could do the job as good as or better than anyone else could. I even volunteered to prove myself to him before he decided. I guess that was the defining point because a few days later I was offered the job. I conquered another fear.

I went into this particular job desiring to learn as much as I could. I never wanted my employer to regret hiring me or to feel cheated in my work performance. I had already learned from previous employers, they didn't want me to be a normal employee, but expected me to be exceptional.

I moved up the corporate ladder quickly. I received raises and promotions and the praise boosted my wounded ego. Not only did I learn how to use the equipment in my office, but I learned how it worked and how to fix it. I did my job and asked for extra work. I had something to prove, not only to my employer, but to myself. I wanted to be both needed and appreciated.

Once all of the challenges were conquered and there was nothing more to prove, I decided to move on. I applied with a similar company with better pay and benefits. When I went for my interview and was told I had to take a typing test I never flinched. Actually, I welcomed the challenge. I was ready to prove my hands were capable.

The interviewer was amazed at my score. While I didn't blow the speed portion of the test away, I did blow the accuracy out of the water. The feeling of triumph was amazing. It had taken me years to learn how to type and I had mastered it. My abilities were well above average. And where I lacked in speed, I made up for in accuracy. In fact, I was told that no one had ever beaten my score on accuracy.

Throughout these jobs, finding and focusing on my strength helped me to overcome my weakness. Confidence is not something you just acquire; it is earned.

Note:
Looking back over this chapter of my life, I realized that I didn't mention God one time. It really bothered me and I wondered why. Then I realized that I questioned the same thing, as I was going through these trails. I felt so alone as if God had just left me. However, now I see that He was carrying me through it all.

God allowed me to go through these things in order to prove to myself that I could. He pushed me to my limits and then showed me how to rise above them. He showed me that He won't just step in and fix our problems, and make them go away, but He will give us the guidance, strength, determination and knowledge to do so. He expects us to do what is possible and leave the impossible to Him.

I can do all things through Christ which strengtheneth me.
                                              -Philippians 4:13

Chapter Nine

The Fairy Tale

> *If ye then, being evil, know how to give good gifts unto your children, how much more shall your Father which is in heaven give good things to them that ask him?*
> -Matthew 7:11

It was one of my biggest fears. Would I ever find my soul mate? Would anyone ever be able to look beyond my imperfections and see the woman underneath the scars? Would I ever find the love like my parents shared? Or would I settle for anything trying to find something?

In all fairness, I dated some amazing guys. Each one holds a very special place in my heart, for their willingness to try to see me as a woman underneath the scars, but none of them managed to accept each aspect of me or give me what I needed. Even though they tried, still I was a burden they didn't have the heart to carry.

Asking someone to share the scars that burdened my life was terrifying. They would have many of the same questions I had, but could or would they accept the fact that there were no answers. I had no choice, but they did. I worried that even if it came to the stages of marriage, would they resent me in the future?

Okay so I'm going to warn you, I'm a hopeless romantic.

Underneath the Scars

I believe God is all-wise. He knew my fears and He knew I would need a helpmate. There was a man born destined to love me, even before I was conceived in my mom's womb. I prayed for him and God sent him to me.

Thanks to a friend and a blind date, I met the man of my dreams; only he turned out to be more than I dreamed possible. Our first date was perfect. We went to the movies and he held my hand. Other guys had held my hand before, but the simple gesture of affection usually prompted twenty questions. I waited, but no questions were asked.

As the dates progressed, I continued to anticipate the usual questions, but they never surfaced - not even in his eyes.

When the day arrived for me to meet his family, I was terrified. Honestly, by this point I believed that perhaps God had answered my prayer. I had asked Him to send me someone that could see the person underneath the scars first and I believed he couldn't see my hands as they were. I was falling in love with him and I was so afraid his family would open his eyes and he would see my imperfections. The thought of him looking at me as a burden he didn't have the heart to carry, terrified me. He held the power to destroy my heart in his hands. Little did I know at the time, but I held his heart in my hands as well.

I tortured myself and didn't give him enough credit. With every date I figured this is it. This will be the date he discovers my imperfections and cuts a trail. And then one day unexpected he picked up my hand, looked at it as if it were really beautiful and kissed it as a valued treasure. From that moment on, I wasn't afraid anymore. He had slain my demons from the past and offered me his unconditional love.

I will never forget how I felt when he slipped the little velvet box out of his pocket. That night underneath the stars, he took my hand in his and asked me to be his forever. As he slipped the diamond ring on my finger my breath caught in my throat and my eyes filled with tears. With all of the people in the world to love, he chose me. He didn't have to love me. There was no family obligation. So many times he could have walked away from me, but he chose to stay. His love for me was real - I could see it in his eyes and feel it in his touch.

While I was so thankful for him and his love, in the back of my mind I thought he deserved better than me. He deserved a woman without scars and an unknown diagnosis. The day I took his last name before God, our family and friends, I knew he would enter the ugliness of my life. People would stare at him and wonder what possessed him to marry a woman with scars. I loved him enough to spare him the heartache, but too much to walk away. I tried to convince myself he would be better off without me. Simply put, he wasn't willing to let me go without a fight.

One year later we were married without him even asking about my hands. We had a simple ceremony at my parent's house with only immediate family. A part of me wanted the church wedding I had always dreamed of, but my fears prevented it from happening. Even after we got our marriage license, I was so afraid he would change his mind. So, I opted to get married at my parent's house that way if he changed his mind, I wouldn't have to suffer the humiliation of standing at the altar with no groom.

Underneath the Scars

The morning of our wedding, I was so nervous. I paced and looked at the clock, counting the minutes until his arrival. When he walked through the door, looking as nervous as I felt, with the grin I loved so much on his face, I knew it would all work out.

It's amazing to me now, how I assumed he would be better off without me in the beginning. At that time, I felt he had given me everything possible with his love and I had nothing significant to offer him in return. Our anniversary usually turned out to be the one occasion when he told me the words in his heart. Usually, I got sappy cards that confessed his undying love that I found absolutely priceless! However, there was one year when he showed me exactly what his heart felt for me. If we live to be old, I don't think he could ever top the Love Plant.

That year, like most, we were poor. I mean *really* poor. He asked me what I wanted, and I knew we couldn't afford anything extravagant, but he was determined to buy me something. So, I suggested a simple houseplant and he agreed.

He worked nightshift at the time, so I knew when he came home from work he would have my present. He woke me up in the wee hours of the morning. As I walked into the living room to see my gift, he was standing there grinning like a fool, thinking he had done something great. I sighed and fought back the tears.

The plant was dead! Brown leaves were lying in the floor around the plant and many more threatened to fall. I tried to sound grateful, but I was mad. I figured he went into the store, grabbed the plant closest to the door, and didn't even notice it was hideous. Then, I felt bad; I thought perhaps he had bought it because it was on clearance. However, the receipt lying on the counter showed he had indeed paid full price.

He had definitely rendered me speechless. I guess the expression on my face, or the withheld thank you, alarmed him and made him question me.

"I thought you wanted a plant," he said, clearly frustrated.

"I did! I wanted a plant with green, shiny leaves. But this one…this one is dead," I said, as my eyes filled with tears.

He sat down on the couch and pulled me into his arms. "When I went into the store all of the other plants were beautiful. I knew someone would buy them, but this one was dying. That's how I felt before I met you. I was dying and your love helped save me. I thought maybe you could save the plant, too," he said.

That was one of the sweetest things anyone had ever said to me. I cried - not tears of sorrow or anger, but tears of joy and thankfulness.

The next day I bought a new container, transplanted it, pruned it and stood back to watch it grow. It was as if it grew right before my eyes. The leaves turned bright green and were shinny. It was the most beautiful plant I had ever seen. Pruning became a weekly chore, and the plant reached the ceiling several times. It was our love plant and it grew just like our love - strong and beautiful. I hope to never forget the love plant and the love that bought it.

Over the next few years, our love bloomed and blossomed and our desire to have children surfaced. All of my fears were still intact, but my husband's love helped to put them at bay. Before I knew it, we were expecting our first child.

The first time I felt the tiny movement, I fell in love and my worries no longer mattered. All I could think about was the precious baby growing inside me - my baby. While we didn't know what waited around the next corner, we were determined to face it as a family and to be thankful however God decided to bless us.

I enjoyed my pregnancy to the fullest. As soon as the first trimester passed, we started picking out names and buying unisex items for the baby.

My obstetrician was wonderful. She never mentioned my hands. Everything was going great and then one day it all changed. I was told at my regular visit I needed to meet with a genetics counselor. All of my fears suddenly returned with a vengeance. I clutched the appointment card in my hand and was terrified of the unknown. I still didn't have a diagnosis for my condition and the 'what ifs' started racing through my mind.

How could I have been so selfish? How could I ask my child to bear the same scars I had lived with? Would my husband ever be able to forgive me? While the thoughts popped in and out of my head, I rubbed my swollen belly and apologized.

Then, I prayed!

I couldn't imagine my child encountering the same hardships I had encountered. I wanted to protect my innocent baby. Finally, when I couldn't take it any longer, I talked to my husband. I explained my qualms with a heart full of tears. He took me in his arms and comforted me with his strength and love.

"We'll face whatever happens. And what are you afraid of, anyway? There's nothing wrong with you!" my husband said.

His words and sincerity touched me. With faith I pressed forward, determined to prevail against the odds. I cancelled my appointment and told my doctor it didn't matter how my child looked - I would love it the same.

When the blessed day arrived, I was no longer scared. The excitement of holding my baby in my arms chased away any doubts. With God's help, I delivered a beautiful baby boy. He had my eyes, and my husband's hands.

I was a little overwhelmed as they handed me my bundle of joy and assumed I knew what to do with him. There was no instruction manual and more fears reared up and plagued me. Sure I had changed my baby doll Sara's diaper countless times, but she didn't move. I could roll her however I wanted and she never complained. But could I change my own baby's diaper? Would I be able to hold him in my arm and feed him at the same time? Could I hold him and bathe him? The thought of not being able to care for my own child worried me. And the thought of failing him in some ways due to my scars, hurt.

At first things were tough. I couldn't hold his legs with one hand and change his diaper with the other, but where there is a will there is a way, as the old saying goes, and I found my own way. Perhaps I was never a pro, but the numerous diapers I changed made me somewhat proficient. I'm not sure his exact age when I stopped carrying the bulb syringe around, fearing he might get choked and my hands would prevent me from helping him, but eventually I relaxed and enjoyed being his mama. Somewhere along the way I realized, while I knew nothing about raising my child, and I was sure to make mistakes, God was always a faith call away. There might be things that come up that I can't handle, due to my hands or not, but there is nothing too big for God.

Underneath the Scars

Holding my precious baby in my arms, watching him grow and discover the world around him made me open my own eyes and look at my life differently. Fear almost cost me that joy and love like I had never felt before. The first time they laid him in my arms and I looked at his tiny face I understood the power of a miracle. I had a better understanding of my parent's feelings the day I was born.

Years later and he thinks he is the lucky one. He thanks God for sending me to him. Because you guessed it, he prayed for someone **SPECIAL** to love. You'd better be careful what you ask for, God just might grant it. He longs to give good gifts to his children, even if it's a fairytale.

Chapter Ten

Tolerance is not Acceptance

So God created man in his own image, in the image of God created he him; male and female created he them.
                                                                -Genesis 1:27

    I had it all figured out. I would sit at my computer and these wonderful words would litter my blank pages with a masterpiece. I would write when the mood struck me and it would be fun. However, it didn't happen that way. I would wake up in the middle of the night with words dancing in my head waiting to be written. Many nights while the world around me slept, I was pouring my heart out onto empty pages. When I would read what I had written, it would frighten me. I didn't want to be so exposed. I didn't want to reveal all of my emotions.

    In truth, I wanted to hide. I had originally thought being a writer would enable me to hide from the world. People would read the black and white pages, the brief biography, and see the picture (of only a headshot) and be none the wiser that I had ABS. It would be an easy way for me to be a coward, and no one would know, except me and God, of course. My family would be thrilled I was following my dreams and they would never question my motivation. I would never have to suffer another interview for employment again.

Underneath the Scars

I jumped right into my first children's book about a zebra with no stripes and was pleased with the finished manuscript (at first, that is). The more I read it, though, the more I realized something was missing, but what? I ignored the whispers of my heart and continued.

I was determined to write books to inspire children to accept themselves regardless of the situation. But the word, ACCEPT, left an uneasy feeling in my pit of my stomach. I tried to shake it off. Of course, I accepted myself, didn't I?

Actually, I didn't! I was just tolerating myself and my situation. I hid behind my scars. I hid my hands as often as I could, and I refused to reveal any scars that sleeves and shoes could hide. However, even though I hid my imperfections, I still knew they remained. Every time I saw a cute sleeveless shirt or sandals, my heart ached for the courage to wear them, but I refused.

And then one day, everything changed. When the woman at the drive-thru gasped in shock at my hand and dropped my change, I was forced to reevaluate my life. I was so appalled the woman could be so cruel that I, in turn, acted just as ugly. While I didn't verbally say anything, the daggers shooting from my eyes said it all. I was furious and I blamed her.

I hated it! I despised all of the stares and whispers that accompanied me around every corner. People where compelled to look at me and pass unfair judgment. I was sentenced to a life of prejudice. As if that weren't already bad enough, I became more self-conscious.

I tossed my children's book in a drawer and decided I didn't want to go down that path after all. It was just too complicated.

Instead, I decided to write a romance novel. My main character was beautiful, with no imperfections. Two years and 80,000 words later, I still wasn't any closer to my dreams. Yes, I was writing, but not what touched my heart. Aggravated and confused, I deleted the manuscript and pulled out my children's book. I was determined to finish his story, yet not sure how.

Then one day unexpectedly, I was enlightened. As I sat in front of the television and watched a video of my son's birthday party, I was shocked. Yes, I knew the woman on the screen – but something was different. I scooted in for a closer look. Even though I remembered doing the things I watched, to actually step back and see it was amazing. And yes, I even STARED!

The woman I saw on the screen wasn't the one I saw in the mirror. I looked handicapped; my elbows curved slightly, one arm was slightly longer than the other, and my scarred hands looked broken, as if they were incapable of doing anything. When my hands completed something that looked truly impossible, but managed to do it anyway – that's where the amazing part kicked in. With my mouth gaped open, I better understood why people had been staring at me.

I knew I couldn't hide anymore; I had to take the next step. I was so tired of always being a victim. I pulled one of my coveted sleeveless shirts from my closet and tried it on. I felt naked and exposed. I quickly pulled it off and hung it back in my closet, all the while, trying to convince myself to wear the stupid shirt. *Just put it on and wear it!* I laid it on my dresser and decided I would wear it to work the next day.

Underneath the Scars

That night I couldn't sleep for thinking about the shirt. I tossed and turned, with the very worst possible scenarios dancing through my head. I'm just glad none of the kids I wanted to help find their own acceptance, witnessed my breakdown.

I almost changed three times before I got to the car, and vowed to turn around and go back home every 500 yards on my way to work. I eased out of the car with butterflies in my stomach while trying to act like nothing was wrong. Inside I was a basket case. *What possessed me to try to find my acceptance anyway?* I questioned. I liked hiding in the shadows, doubting and wallowing in self-pity. Didn't I?

I was defenseless and exposed while everyone starred. As they talked to me, their eyes drifted to my scarred arm. I wanted to cry and throw a temper tantrum. I almost faked an illness to go home. Right before I decided to throw in the towel, my wonderful determination kicked in.

I lifted my stubborn chin a few notches and ignored it all. *Fine let them all stare if it makes them feel better.* Then I remembered that these wonderful people were my friends. It was a shock to them because I had hid it for so long.

Somehow, I made it through the day, despite the several promises to myself, to destroy the stupid, heartbreaking, sleeveless shirt when I got home.

Once I entered my safe haven, I broke into sobs. I allowed all the heartache, pushed aside all day, to surface. I cried until it was all released. And when I was finished, it all didn't seem as devastating as it had only moments prior.

The next day, I donned another sleeveless shirt and repeated the previous day. I continued the process until I could put on a sleeveless shirt without breaking out in a sweat. Now, open toed shoes were an entirely different matter. I would go into a shoe store and try on all the wonderful sandals. I would look in the mirror and pray for the strength to wear them, but the fear remained.

Finally one day it happened. I gathered enough courage to buy the cutest pink sandals. I clutched them to my chest on the way to the counter to pay for them. I nearly jumped out of my skin when the clerk appeared and asked me if there was anything else I needed. I half expected her to laugh at me or tell me to put them back. Instead, she tucked them in a bag and told me to have a nice day.

I sat in the parking lot at work, trying to gain the courage to wear the shoes, instead of only admiring them. I took out the shoes and slipped them on. They were so much cuter than the shoes I was wearing. A few tears and prayers later, I got out of the car and forced myself to go inside. I walked quickly as if I had something to hide. I hurriedly placed my feet under my desk and smiled.

I WAS WEARING SANDALS!!

Later when I had forgotten about my sandals, I turned around, crossed my legs, and started talking to several of my co-workers. I noticed a few of them looking at my feet. The anxiety bubbled. The tears welled. And I took control. I smiled and thought perhaps they liked my new sandals as much as I did. I was determined to show the world the woman underneath the scars.

As I continued to brave new attire, I also continued to work on my picture book about Zippy the zebra. Each draft showed me more of the direction I wanted to go, but it was still far away from where I wanted to be. Likewise, in my heart, I knew I was headed in the right direction with my life. I had surpassed tolerance and was headed for acceptance of myself.

Chapter Eleven

Stares and Smiles

A merry heart doeth good like a medicine: but a broken spirit drieth the bones.
                                                    -Proverbs 17:22

If I had a nickel for every time some asked me - What happened to your hands, arm or foot? - or made a rude comment about my scars, then I wouldn't need to work anymore. If I had a nickel for every time someone's eyes darted to my scars and lingered, then I would have more money than I could spend in this lifetime. I'd be able to retire on a private villa somewhere tropical and laze on the white sand all day.

Not everyone intends to make me feel uncomfortable. It is kind of like going by a car wreck; they try to look away but are compelled to stare anyway. To be honest, I've unintentionally stared at people myself. We all have, and to say you haven't would be like saying you're perfect.

So, why do people stare, anyway?

Some stare out of ignorance. Those are the same people who laugh and smirk at my scars. They are rude and simply don't care about other people's feelings. They have their own physical or mental limitations and to see someone else scarred makes them feel better about themselves. In my experience, they have often been the victims of teasing and staring themselves.

Some stare out of sympathy. They are genuinely concerned. They want to know what happened and why. They worry and perhaps even pray when they see someone hurt or scarred. It is their nature to care.

Some stare out of amazement. They can't believe what their eyes are actually seeing so they look again, just as I did when I saw myself on the video. We all love to see the impossible turn into the possible. I once read about Jim Abbott and how crowds of people would gather into the stadiums to watch the so-called handicapped pitcher play professional baseball. They would watch him play for innings not realizing it was actually him because his performance was superb. We are often not what people expect us to be, so they stare in awe.

So what's the secret to handling situations when people stare?

It has happened to everyone over the course of his or her life. You notice someone staring at you and immediately feel awkward and uncomfortable. So how do you handle these situations?

Take control, first and foremost of the situation. Whenever we are in control of a situation, it makes us feel better and ultimately handle it wiser. Look at the person and acknowledge them with a smile and then resume whatever you were doing. If you act nervous or fidget, shove your hands in your pockets (which is what I used to do), or try to hide your scars, the person staring is in control of you. Usually, a smile will nip it in the bud, but if they proceed to stare, ignore them. While we can't control other people's actions, we can control our own. Staring back at them or showing any kind of displeasure feeds their curiosity and rudeness.

If they make a comment, assess the situation. Why are they asking; it is out of concern, amazement, or just plain ignorance? Generally, you can tell by the person's body language and tone of voice. If it seems they are concerned and intrigued by me, I will explain my condition and answer their questions. If they seem rude and ignorant, I ignore them with as much friendliness as possible. I don't allow people to put their hands on me or make me feel uncomfortable. No one EVER has the right to treat people badly just because they aren't considered the norm. The way I see it they are the one with the problem, not me. If they persist, I walk away or politely reprimand them. You'd be surprised at how a stern yet nice voice can get a point across. However, I never lower myself to their behavior. I always treat others the way I want them to treat me, not as they have treated me.

When they say – Oh, poor you! – I give them my best smile; the one that reaches my eyes and makes my face glow. I respond by saying something like, "Actually, I'm thankful to be alive! I could have died, but yet I'm alive to love and be loved. These scars remind me daily that I am a survivor."

Usually, that will stop their pity. It makes them stop and evaluate their own lives. They wonder how I can be so thankful when I am burdened with scars. Why do I see myself as a survivor instead of a victim? I believe it gives them hope for their own life. That's where the word inspiration comes from. Some people look at being an inspiration to others as being bad, but to me, it's wonderful. Anytime my life can inspire another life by offering them hope is a great blessing. It means I didn't give up and quit when I often felt like doing just that. It means I am persevering, living my dreams, and defeating my own fears. I want to make a difference!

However, I'm not always strong. One day while my kids were on summer break from school, I had a meeting. While we were waiting, the kids across from us noticed my hands, stared, and laughed. For the first time, in such a long time, anger reared up and slapped me in the face. I was defenseless against the rude behavior. It didn't bother me that they had treated me so cruel, but that my children were there. I wanted to rant and rave, but little eyes were on me. We can tell our children a hundred times how to handle a situation, but sometimes we just need to show them.

I held up my head, looked the children in the eyes (the ones laughing and being so cruel) and smiled at them. I challenged them with my eyes and smile. They looked away and their laughter subsided. I actually felt pity for them. In my eyes, they had been neglected and not taught how to be kind and considerate of others.

I wanted to protect my kids from the cruel reality of my life. That's the hardest part for me when someone I love is affected by the way others react to my scars. Panicked I searched their faces for backlash of the situation, and they seemed fine. They did comment, however, on how ugly the kids acted.

There are times when it doesn't bother me at all for people to stare, and then there are days when I just don't feel strong enough to handle it, times when I feel like I could stand before the whole world, and times when it's hard to face myself.

Recently, I was attending my son's first grade Easter party. While we were waiting in line, a little boy walked up to me and asked me about my arm. It was one of those bad days when the questions were bound to send me over the edge. I began my usual child explanation, "I was born this way." I didn't expect it to stop there, it never does. I looked at my son to see whether he was bothered by the conversation. My mind was racing, trying to figure out a way to stop the situation before it affected him. Before I had a chance to do or say anything more, he picked up my hand and covered it with his. Then he placed my hand against his face. It was as if he was showing the child, there was nothing wrong with his mama. The questions stopped and I knew God had intervened.

Thankfully, I don't always see when people stare at me. I believe God shelters us from it many times. For example, once I was in the pharmacy when the cashier asked to speak to me privately. She looked aggravated as we walked to the side, away from the counter. She said, "Do people always stare at you?" I didn't realize what she was asking me, until she explained that the woman beside me was staring at my hands and smirking. Honestly, I didn't even notice the woman.

We all desire to feel accepted, loved, accomplished, and cherished. We all want to be happy. So, what makes us happy?

For me, happiness is not one thing, but many combined. I feel so blessed to find joy in something as simple as a smile or a flower bursting with a colorful bloom. Isn't it funny how we look at flowers and just expect them to be beautiful? We take their beauty for granted and never stop to think of the hardships faced along the way. Have you ever seen one flower standing among the weeds and wondered how it got there? To our eyes, it just seems out of place, but perhaps it was because it was the only flower strong enough to survive the weeds.

Underneath the Scars

While other people can add to our happiness, no one can make us happy. That is a choice we make. A great job, material possessions, or people won't help if we decide in our hearts to be miserable.

Every day we open our eyes and take a breath is a gift from God, and I intend to treat it that way. I work hard (probably harder than most), but I do it because it needs to be done. I'm thankful that I didn't settle for the life I was expected to have, but struggled to find the one I wanted to live.

Regardless of battles I face daily – I'm happy!

Living with scars has helped me look beyond the exterior of everything and see the beauty underneath it all. I'm able to look past the ugly looks and comments and smile.

Chapter Twelve

Out of the Mouths of Kids

Out of the mouth of babes and sucklings hast thou ordained strength because of thine enemies, that thou mightest still the enemy and the avenger.
-Psalm 8:2

    It amazes me at how when we serve God totally in our hearts, there is nothing out of reach. There has always been a desire in my heart to be a teacher, but I never managed to open that door. As I said earlier, I couldn't afford to go back to school and the way was never made for me to pursue that avenue of my life. Of course, like many, I could have opted for student loans, but there were still always obstacles I couldn't overcome. This is just another example of God's plan for me and how He has blessed my life.

    Around the time I was denied funding to further my education to be a teacher, God gave me the gift to teach Sunday school at church. While I don't have the required qualifications to teach at a school administered by the state, God gave me everything I would need to teach children about Him – the most important part of life.

    I was a little hesitant, at first, because I didn't know much about the scriptures. I couldn't go deep into the Bible and explain it the way most teachers can. I felt inadequate because I didn't feel like I had what it took to be a Sunday school teacher. And then God showed me the most important quality, love. He placed a love so deep in my heart for those children; I can't even explain how wonderful it is.

There is nothing as beautiful as hearing children's voices recite the Lord's Prayer or sing Jesus Loves Me. There is such joy in seeing their little eyes light up with the power of understanding. It pleases my heart tremendously to place a little sticker beside their name each Sunday for their dedication in coming to church. And just to know that I am teaching them something so important, that they will take with them throughout their whole lives, humbles me.

However, it didn't take me long to understand that they were teaching me, too.

One little boy questioned everything I said. He wouldn't just sit quietly and listen; he always wanted to know more. So one day as I was teaching, he asked me, "If God created the Heavens and the earth, then who created God."

I replied, "I don't know. My Bible starts with 'In the beginning God created...' That's as far back as I can go. God is a Spirit and has always existed."

My answer obviously didn't satisfy him because he continued to ask more questions. It unnerved me that I couldn't answer his questions to his satisfaction. Finally, I said, "Go ask your dad." (His dad was the adult Sunday school teacher.)

He looked at me in the eyes and smiled as he said, "I did, already, and he told me what you said."

I could have been aggravated that he had put me through such torture, but I was so relieved that I had at least answered the question okay. And because he literally questioned everything I said, it made me study more and try harder.

There were two little boys who walked alone to church each Sunday. Talk about touching my heart. They came because they wanted to, not because someone made them. I often wondered whether I would have had that kind of dedication as a child, and I can honestly say that I wouldn't have. I don't think I would have put down my toys to walk to church and sit quietly and listen when I could have been playing. The fact that they do, touches my heart in a way I can't even explain. These boys taught me a lesson about going to church out of obligation versus going out of desire.

Working from home and taking care of two children, especially during the summer is tough. There was one day I was trying to meet a deadline and I was really feeling the pressure. The kids kept interrupting me, and finally, I snapped. I yelled, screamed, cried, and felt overwhelmed by it all. A little later, my oldest son came up to me and asked, "Mama, I know we're supposed to put God first in our lives, but I forget what comes next?"

I couldn't help but smile as I replied, "Our family and then our job." The words hit my heart before they hit my ears.

Talk about getting my words thrown in my face. He helped me get to my priorities straight. I realized my kids were more important than my job. Instead of feeling overwhelmed by it all, I just needed to ask God to help me. I learned to get up earlier and get my work done before they woke or take advantage of the time they were busy watching their favorite shows. I also started taking them to the park and I worked in the shade while they played. If we look to Him, God will always provide us a way.

Sometimes when we are doing something, it's hard at the time to see any results and we tend to assume we aren't making any progress. My pastor tells me, "You're doing better than what you think." More often than not, I have found this statement to be so true in my life. We tend to get discouraged when the accomplishments are not immediate and fail to remember that some things take time.

I was feeling discouraged and wondered whether my time of teaching was coming to an end. I couldn't seem to keep their attention long enough to tell a story, and then I wondered when I finished, if they even heard or understood a word I had said. I asked God to help me. I felt like I was stalled at a crossroad and I honestly didn't know which way to go. Then God answered my prayer. One of the kids in my Sunday school class had asked his mom if Teacher (that's what he called me) was like God. She explained to him that God lived in my heart. He replied, "Then I like God." When I heard this, I realized I was doing better than what I had originally thought. I had made a difference in this child's life and wasn't that the whole purpose?

Sometimes we just don't give kids enough credit. We assume because they are small that they can't do or understand the things we can. I had decided to teach the kids to recite the Lord's Prayer. Since I have all ages of children in Sunday school, I had different levels. The older kids had to recite it to me, the younger kids had to read it, and the smaller ones had to repeat it after me, in order to get an accomplishment certificate.

Candida Sullivan

    I was practicing at home with my oldest son who was eight at the time. He was reciting and struggling. When he got to a part he didn't know, my younger son, who was four, jumped in and helped him. My mouth gapped open as I turned and looked at him. He started from the beginning and said the whole prayer without missing a word. I was shocked. And then he said, "I know them commandments, too."

    Throughout the years, I've come to appreciate innocent, yet profound wisdom, which comes from the mouths of children.

Underneath the Scars

Chapter Thirteen

Ability in Disability

For I have learned, in whatever state I am, therewith to be content.
-Philippians 4:11

In another person's eyes, I'm handicapped, disabled, defective, special, a miracle, an angel, etc. But in my eyes, I'm just me.

When other people see me as being disabled, I see that I'm able. When they see me as being handicapped, I see that I'm able to find my own way of doing anything that I truly want to do. When they see me as being defected, I see that I survived. When they see me as being special, a miracle, or angel, I see that I am so blessed!

One day, unexpectedly I was asked to attend Career Day at my children's school. I was thrilled and terrified, at the same time. Not only would I stand before tons of kids, but I would be reading my story about a little zebra with no stripes, which would, in turn, raise questions about my own scars. Even though I was thrilled with the opportunity, still the fear almost unnerved me. I wanted to hide my scars as best as I could, but I refused to go back down that road. For others attending Career Day, it would be solely about their careers; for me it would also involve my scars. (Not to mention I had social anxiety. Just the thought of hundreds of little eyes staring at my scars all at once terrified me. My whole body trembled.)

Underneath the Scars

I was nearly ready to escape and go home where I planned to hide under the covers for the remainder of the day, when God gave me the courage I needed to stay. I talked to a teacher outside and was told to be myself and everyone would love me. After a few deep breaths and a silent prayer, I entered the building.

When the teacher introduced me to the kids as a children's author, I felt like a fraud. Yes, I spent my days and most of my nights writing children's books and stories, but I had never been published. I didn't feel like I had earned the title of author, yet. To me it was more of a dream that I was striving for, but hadn't accomplished.

I could tell them what it was like to write a book. I had done that many times. I could tell them what it was like to chase a dream for years that seemed so far out of reach. I could tell them how hard it was to blend the words together to make a story. But I couldn't tell them what it was like to hold in my hands a book I had written or to see the story come to life with illustrations.

I could tell them what it felt like for one publisher to say yes, and then not being able to go through with it. I could tell them all about rejections. In fact, I could show them hundreds of rejection letters.

Instead of all of the negative aspects, I decided to encourage them to dream, and to believe in those dreams until they came true. No, my dreams hadn't come true yet, but I had faith that they would. Sometimes I believe it makes more of an impact on people, when they watch you struggle to be successful, rather than when you've already achieved success.

I stood in front of the kids with my heart and scars exposed and read them my story about Zippy the zebra. I addressed my scars and answered their questions. It wasn't just about a zebra with no stripes, but how not having stripes made him feel. His feelings were my feelings, and in all reality, that little zebra was me. I hated the vulnerability and felt nervous. My throat was dry and my heart pounded. I wanted to be a coward and run away. Was it ironic that my answer was inside the very book I had written to help children overcome being different?

When I first started writing about Zippy, I hoped it would help at least one person overcome the obstacles in their way. As I lifted my head, squared my shoulders and looked over the crowd of smiling children, I realized that the first person that book helped was me.

I read my book, answered their questions, and encouraged them to believe in their own dreams. Some cried, some hugged me, and most smiled, I walked away feeling indescribable. Regardless of the success I find in my life, I don't know if anything could ever compare to the way I felt surrounded by children, watching the expressions on their faces as I read them one of my stories. No amount of money could ever compare to how I felt in that moment. Even though, it was unpublished and there were no illustrations to accompany the words, they still enjoyed it. I've often wondered whether the message of treating others the way we want to be treated impacted their lives in any way. I wonder when they are teasing other children with differences, if they can see me standing before them with scarred hands, reading them a story about how it feels to be teased.

The next day, I walked my children into school, as I had numerous times, but it was different. I was no longer just a parent. *I was the storyteller.* For the remainder of the year, I was blessed each morning with waves and smiles and invitations to come back again. Kids continue to approach me in restaurants and grocery stores, while their parents tell me they've heard all about me.

That day I volunteered my time to tell children all about what it's like to be a writer and was blessed without measure. I found my ability instead of disability.

Chapter Fourteen

The Choice to be Happy

Be glad in the LORD, and rejoice, ye righteous: and shout for joy, all ye that are upright in heart.
                                                            -Psalm 32:11

    Wouldn't it be great if we could be happy every day without any heartaches or problems? If we could breeze through every day with smiles and laughs and tears were forgotten. What kind of person would we be? Would we really be happy?

    In my experience, everything that comes easy isn't necessarily appreciated. Often times, it's the challenge of the battle that makes the victory so sweet. If I bounced out of bed each morning with a smile on my face, no struggles to deal with and no accomplishments to strive for, then what would be the point? If everything, including happiness, was handed to me, then I would be spoiled. I would come to expect it and never really appreciate the greatness of it. I believe in life, it's not the struggles we overcome that inspires others, but it's the way we overcome our struggles.

    When I got married, someone told me to appreciate the bad times. At the time, it didn't make any sense to me. Who in the world appreciates bad times? However, now I understand that statement. Someone who has never been sad cannot truly appreciate being happy. Someone who has never been poor cannot truly appreciate wealth. Someone who has never been sick cannot truly appreciate good health. If we've never been weak then how can we appreciate strength?

I love the opportunities in my life when the tears roll down my face. Those tears help me to grow as a person. The ability to cry means: I love, I hurt, I forgive, I sympathize, I hope, I dream, I'm disappointed, I'm weak, I'm happy, I'm determined, and most of all - I'm alive.

There have been many times in my life when it felt like I was stranded in a deep dark hole with no way out. Rather than trying to find my way out, it would have been easier to give up. Regardless of how dark life gets, I'm so thankful I can always find a spark of hope. As long as I'm alive there's hope that things will get better. If you look in the mirror every day and don't like the reflection starring back you - then do something to change it. You are the only person who can make a difference in your life.

I used to get up every morning, squeeze into my clothes and think: I need to go on a diet. Yet, I didn't. I complained and stressed about my weight every day, instead of doing something to change it. I was miserable.

Finally, overwhelmed and thoroughly discouraged, I decided to make a change. Wow, <u>it was hard</u>! I stopped eating sugar and potato chips. (I loved potato chips!) I forced myself to exercise at least three times a week. At first, I thought I would die. I hated all of the health foods and exercise videos. I was hungry and sore. Nevertheless, I refused to give up. The pounds came off, albeit slowly. One to two pounds a week was all I could manage to lose.

Every week got a little easier. I started trying new recipes and actually looked forward to my exercise routine. When clothes that I hadn't fit into in years finally fit again, I was so proud of myself. I learned to set realistic goals and meet them. I enjoyed making healthier selections and educating myself of healthier living. Although I fell off the wagon many times, if not weekly, I didn't stay there.

My point is this: losing weight was something I had to do for myself. No one could force me. It was something I desired to do in my heart and that's why I was able to achieve it. Do I miss eating candy bars, real potato chips, and fast food? Nah! Occasionally, I treat myself, but for the most part, I don't miss it at all.

Other difficult times have mostly been associated with my great ability to procrastinate. Why do today what we can do tomorrow, right?

Well, I've learned that eventually tomorrow comes and then we're overwhelmed. I was so bad to put things off. If I needed to accomplish a task, I would lay it aside and think about it every day. I dreaded it, and with each passing day, dreaded it more. My arsenal comprised several excuses:

- I'll do it later
- I don't feel like doing anything right now
- I feel bad
- I'm tired
- I'll just rest for a while and do everything this evening
- I work better under pressure

Underneath the Scars

All of these excuses became my famous quotes, and I never seemed to get anything accomplished. My house was dirty, my work piled to the ceiling, and I didn't know how to get out of the hole I had dug for myself. I didn't want to acknowledge that the first step was recognizing the problem and wanting to fix it.

Realizing it would be one task at a time helped to get started. I understood that I didn't get in this shape overnight and thus wasn't going to be able to fix it with the snap of my fingers. I couldn't just clean my house, organize my office, and promise to do better. I had to change my way of doing things and make myself do them every day.

There is nothing like having a list of accomplishments at the end of every day. Likewise, happiness is not handed to anyone - it is achieved. If you want to be happy then you have to work toward being happy. We can't just roll out of bed every morning and say, "Okay, God. I'm awake. Bless me now." It doesn't quite work that way. God will bless us every single day, in fact, just being alive is a blessing, but the harder we work at it, the happier we can be.

Every morning when I wake up, I realize that I have two choices: I can either be happy or be miserable. I can have a good day or a bad day. When things happen in my life and get me down, I can either label myself as a victim or strive to be a survivor. Have you ever met someone who is always a victim? Everything bad that happens in their life is someone else's fault. They never take responsibility for their own actions. They blame everyone else for their misery, but never realize they have the power to change their own attitude. I've often heard throughout my life that a positive attitude is half the battle. As for me, I *choose* to be happy despite my circumstance.

Chapter Fifteen

Mold Me Lord

But now, O LORD, thou art our father; we are the clay, and thou our potter; and we all are the work of thy hand.
                                                               -Isaiah 64:8

For as long as I can remember, I've always wondered why God chose me to bear these scars that will last a lifetime. In my worst days, I've been heartbroken, ashamed, and immersed in self-pity. It was during these times, I believed God had cursed me, He was mad at me, or perhaps He had forsaken me. There was even a time when I wondered how God could truly love me, and yet, still do something like this to me. After all, He knew from the beginning that I would have a hard time in life, that I would cry myself to sleep at night, withdraw from my family, and become the object of stares and whispers my whole life.

Other times, I've been very angry at God. I would scream from the inside - *WHY? How could you do this to me? What did I do to deserve this?*

In calmer times, I've asked because I was curious. I simply wanted to know why me. Of all of people, why was I the one chosen? (Not that I ever wanted anyone else to bear my scars, but it was always just a question dancing in my mind.)

And then finally, after I come to terms with it all, I've asked with thankfulness. When I no longer believed I was cursed, but blessed, I wondered why God would be so merciful and give me such a beautiful reminder that He spared my life and has a purpose for me.

Success doesn't come without heartaches, compromises and sacrifices - not to mention hard work. Nor does it come without patience. I know from experience. It comes when we allow God to shape us into a vessel He can use.

When the desire to become a published author emerged, I jumped in with both feet without even testing the waters first. By the time I realized what it took to be a published author; I was already to the point of no turning back.

Six years later, it was hard to sit down and write when I hadn't profited financially at all. It was difficult to listen to my heart when my mind was screaming for me to go the other direction.

There was one day when I got up, so sure this would be *the* day. I showered, dressed, and looked forward to the phone call or email I was sure to receive. I shoved my cell phone in my pocket and checked my email every five minutes. But as the hours passed by my hope diminished.

The make-up I had so carefully applied that morning, in hopes that we would be celebrating soon, washed down my face. I stood out on the deck, so the kids wouldn't hear me, and cried. My faith was definitely shaken. I felt like a failure.

I grieved for all the kids I wanted to help, all of the times I was rejected, the little girl who begged God to heal her hands, and I honestly felt like I couldn't do it anymore. I couldn't keep writing. Who was I kidding anyway? The thought of never writing again, living without hopes and dreams, and losing the zeal to help others hurt much worse.

I thought about the story of Moses. He received a death sentence before he was ever born. Like me, though, he was spared. He survived when so many died. God had a plan for Moses before he was ever born. He had an important job for Moses to do - a job only Moses could do. Like me too, Moses had many excuses why he couldn't do the job given to him. But every time Moses gave God and excuse, God gave him a solution. God molded Moses into what He wanted him to be and I know in my heart that's exactly what God was doing with me. God will see me through this journey, one day at a time, the good days as well as the bad. His hands are on me with each turn of the potter's wheel. I have the marks to prove it.

The day when I sat in the doctor's office and was told there was a chance I would be disabled soon, almost destroyed me. It's amazing to me how quickly life can change. One minute I was sitting in an examination room with hope that I would be prescribed some type of medication that would cure my pain, and in the next instant, the rug had been jerked right out from under me.

I managed to stumble out of the office without crying. I unlocked my car as usual and slid behind the wheel. Somehow, I managed to get home with my eyes still dry. I called my family and relayed the doctor's prognosis without shedding a tear.

I had worked my whole life, determined to show the world I was not disabled, and, yet, my determination and hard work were the factors now contributing to my condition. I continued to go through the motions of life for that day; I cooked, cleaned, and helped the kids with their homework. When everything was finished and they were playing, I crawled into bed and pulled the covers over my head.

The events of the day flashed before me. And all I could think was, why God? How could I go into a school, read my books, and inspire anyone if I was receiving a disability check and in constant pain? Why did I have to go through all of the trials and tribulations if this is how my story was going to end?

The next morning, I got up and tried to find my determination and hope once more. I refused to lie in the bed and feel sorry for myself. The pain attacked almost the moment my feet hit the floor. The effort just to take a shower and get dressed was tough. I opened my Bible, hoping God would give me hope. I turned to the scripture God had given me when He gave me the gift to write.

And in that instant, I knew this was just another obstacle I would have to face. It wasn't over for me. While I might not be able to perform the jobs of the world, I could do the things, which God laid on my heart.

Tragedy was averted thanks to the Lord's hands working through twelve weeks of chiropractic care. Once again, He was shaping me for my purpose.

Chapter Sixteen

Trusting the Lord

For ye have need of patience, that, after ye have done the will of God, ye might receive the promise.
-Hebrews 10:36

    I don't think we are ever content. When I was younger, I wanted to be older, and then once I got older I wished I could relive those carefree moments of my youth again, but it was too late. I can remember being at work and thinking about all of the things that I needed to do at home, but once I got home, I thought about all of the things I needed to do at work. When I was pregnant I couldn't wait to see and hold my precious baby, then I couldn't wait for him to take his first step, and utter his first words and, now as they grow older, I long to go back to those moments when I felt them kick in my swollen belly.

    We are never just satisfied with the moment we are currently living in. I know there will be a day when I will wish with my whole heart that I could relive this very moment. This evening at supper, my son irritated me with his fits of giggling. I wanted him to stop, be quiet and eat like everyone else. But it now occurs to me, that one day I could be sitting alone, eating my supper in total silence, and wishing to hear his laughter.

    My biggest problem is I don't have enough patience. I want what I want, right now. No, that isn't entirely correct, I wanted it yesterday. I don't like to struggle with anything and I always seem to want the instant gratification.

If I plant flower seeds today, I want to see beautiful foliage and blooms tomorrow, but I often forget the real beauty is in the nurturing and waiting. I know this because when I walk into a nursery filled with flowers, I don't feel anything. But when I walk into my yard and see all of the beautiful flowers that I planted, nurtured, and anticipated to bloom, it touches me.

It's the same way with prayers. Actually, I wanted the prayer answered before I even prayed. But, I've learned sometimes it takes a while for me to get to the point where I can really pray and then it takes faith and patience for my prayer to be answered.

For ten years, I prayed for my husband to get saved and go to church with me. It was so hard to get up on Sunday mornings and take my children to church, alone. There were so many times when it all seemed hopeless. I got discouraged and wanted to give up. Now, I realize it took me ten years to be able to pray for him because, at first, I wanted him to go to church for me. It took me a long time to get to the point to really desire it in my heart for him.

It's been the same way with this book and my life in general. I wanted the instant success. I didn't want to go through the process. I've had to give up my thoughts and plans and replace them with God's. His timing is perfect.

Some people laugh at me for having faith and trusting God with my life. They think just because God doesn't answer me right away means that there is no God or I've done something wrong. They don't understand that God does all things in His time according to His purpose. We can't give God ultimatums or tell Him to do anything, but He hears the groaning of our hearts. Anytime we insert the word "if" when we are referring to God shows unbelief.

I believe it takes patience and trust to reach our full potential. We have to open our eyes and believe in our hearts God will see us through each trial. We have to strive to be a good person. We have to stop making excuses for our wrong choices, stop and evaluate our lives when it seems they are falling apart, and look to God for guidance.

I know God will bless the hearts of those while they read this book, and it will have nothing to do with me. Any wisdom or knowledge gleaned from this text comes from God.

You are reading this book, because I never gave up. Through it all God showed me about faith, determination, obedience, love, patience, trials and tribulations, heartaches, failures, perseverance, grace, mercy, trust, and that dreams do come true.

My ability to overcome obstacles throughout my life transpired in parallel with the fulfillment of purpose in my life. To be an overcomer takes one simple action: to trust in the Lord with all your heart and know that His thoughts are higher than yours. He has plans for us – not plans to harm us, but plans to prosper us and give us a future.

Trust Him today!

May God bless you always!

Underneath the Scars

FOR KIDS

If I could sit down with all of the kids in the world with Amniotic Band Syndrome or other similar conditions, this is what would I tell them.

Being different isn't always easy; sometimes it's really hard. There were times as a little girl when I prayed for different hands, a time when I really hated my hands. People laughed at me and made me feel bad; they hurt my feelings and I would cry. Sometimes when I was in school, I couldn't do things like other kids. I had to learn to do things my own way. I learned how to overcome the stares and laughs.

What to do when people stare at you.

When I notice someone staring at my hands, I look at them and SMILE. That lets them know I'm a nice person and that I have feelings too. If they continue staring and laughing at me, I look deep into their eyes and smile, and then I walk away. I never act the same way they do. I don't laugh at them, yell or call them names. I don't hit them or give them dirty looks. Why? Just because they're being rude to me doesn't mean I should be rude too. I believe we should always treat others the way we want to be treated (not the way they treat us).

Finding your own way!

Just because I can't do things like other people doesn't mean I can't find my own way of doing things. I write, pick up things, hold things, and do almost everything differently from other people.

Underneath the Scars

Sometimes it comes natural to me and other times I have to really think about it. But overall, I have learned I can do anything I really want to do and you can, too. Sometimes we have to try new ways until we find the way that works the best for us. Even though certain things, like playing sports, piano, typing, etc., are challenging, they are not impossible. If you find something you really want to do – don't give up until you accomplish it.

We are all different!

No one is perfect, so they shouldn't expect us to be perfect either. We all have flaws and differences. That's what makes everyone unique. Some people have blue eyes, some brown; some people are tall, while some are short; some people wear glasses, while others don't. We are all special! God loves each person the same. Never allow anyone to make you feel bad about yourself. We are all beautiful, especially when we take time to see the people underneath it all. When people meet you they might forget what color hair you had, but I bet they would remember your smile. Why? Because smiles make people feel good. Our appearance will soon be forgotten, but kindness is treasured and remembered.

Overcome fear with hope!

I believe as long as we have hope, we can accomplish anything. There were many times in my life that I allowed the fear of failure to prevent me from doing something I really wanted to do. But, I'm not afraid anymore. Of course, I'm not going to be good at everything, but as long as I try, anything is possible. If I'm too afraid to at least try then, guess what? I'm definitely going to fail. I would rather try and fail, than fail because I refused to try. There is always that great possibility that I will succeed. I have hope in my heart and that hope helps me to follow my dreams. I always wanted to be an author. There were many times when I almost gave up because it was hard, but I continued trying and eventually I succeeded.

Just be you!

There is something very special that makes you – you! You don't have to be a hero or try to be someone you're not. People will like you because you're funny or serious, kind, fun to be around, sweet, sincere; the list goes on and on. If you pretend to be someone you're not then you deny people the opportunity to know the real you. Just because my friend likes chocolate cake doesn't mean I have to like it, too. Perhaps I like vanilla cake. Both are really good, and there is no right or wrong answer. Don't ever be afraid to be yourself. You're great just the way you are!

Check out the book *Zippy and the Stripes of Courage* to read about a zebra who didn't look like the others.

Underneath the Scars

ABOUT AMNIOTIC BAND SYNDROME

Amniotic Band Syndrome (ABS) is a rare condition caused by string-like bands in the amniotic sac. These bands can entangle the umbilical cord or other parts of the baby's body. The constriction can cause a variety of problems depending on where they are located and how tightly they are wrapped. The complications from ABS vary. Mild banding can result in amputation or scarring, while severe banding can result in death of the baby.

The medical community cannot truly explain what causes amniotic bands to form. While some call it a fluke of nature, I believe it is a symbol of God's amazing miracles. God doesn't punish us with scars; He blesses us with life. The scars show the world that there is a God and He is great.

Special links and groups for Amniotic Band Syndrome

- http://www.amnioticbandsyndrome.com
- http://health.groups.yahoo.com/group/ABS_support/
- http://www.reach.org.uk/reachcms/
- http://www.helpinghandsgroup.org/
- http://limbdifferences.org/
- http://www.superhands.us/
- http://www.clubfootclub.org/
- http://www.ontheotherhand.org/
- http://www.kidscanplay.com/
- http://www.unlimbitedpossibilities.org/index.html
- http://health.groups.yahoo.com/group/SammysFriends/

ACKNOWLEDGEMENTS

I would like to thank God, foremost – the center of my life. My God exemplifies everything wonderful, beautiful, great, and loving in my life. He blessed me with the vision for this book. Thank you God, for being so wonderfully patient with me, as I fought and struggled against your plan for me. Thank you helping me find acceptance and for showing me that I'm a survivor of Amniotic Band Syndrome. And most of all, thank you for loving me and allowing me to live. Thank you God, for giving me scars to remind me of your great love and mercy just for me and my life.

I have learned that it takes many people to write and complete just one book. In my experience, there were many tears and prayers needed to complete Underneath the Scars. God blessed me with some amazingly strong people to help me along this journey. I would love to take a moment and thank them for their prayers, kindness, love, and support. Without them, none of this would be possible.

Thank you to ALL of my family and friends who encourage me, support me, believe in me, and love me. You will never know how much you mean to me! I decided not to list names on the premise that I might miss someone; however, I hope you know how grateful I am to have you in my life.

I feel so blessed to have worked with the wonderful people at ShadeTree Publishing. They exceeded my expectations on every level. Thank you for your kindness, this wonderful opportunity, and

Underneath the Scars

for believing in me. I could not have asked for a better publishing experience. You all are amazing!

ABOUT THE AUTHOR

Candida Sullivan believes in miracles. She was born with a rare condition called Amniotic Band Syndrome, which generally causes death in most babies before they are ever born. She knows that it a beautiful blessing she survived and wants to show the world that her scars are not a punishment, but instead are a wonderful expression exemplifying God's love and mercy for her life. She believes God spared her for a reason and wants to spend her life telling of the hope and love God placed inside of her.

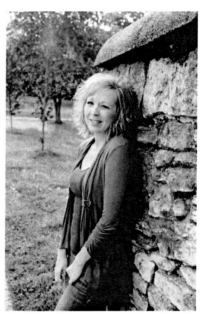

Candida lives in Tennessee with her husband Shannon and two boys, Cayden and Jordon. She teaches Sunday school and loves to be surrounded by the wonder and excitement of kids.

Underneath the Scars

See Candida's children book, *Zippy and the Stripes of Courage,* for a story about how Zippy, who like Candida, came to accept himself.

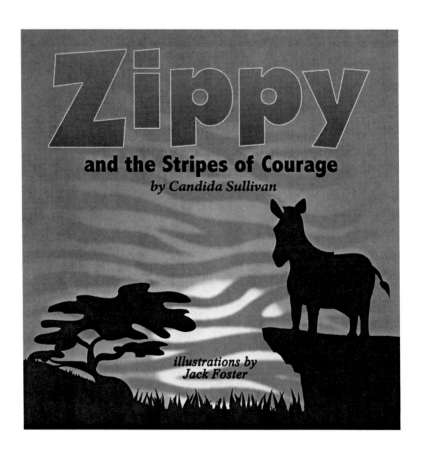

CPSIA information can be obtained at www.ICGtesting.com
Printed in the USA
LVOW111559191111

255740LV00002B/1/P